Preventing Falls

Edited by J. Thomas Hutton, M.D., Ph.D.,
Jeffrey W. Elias, Ph.D.,
JoAnn Leavey Shroyer, Ph.D.,
and Zane Curry, Ph.D.

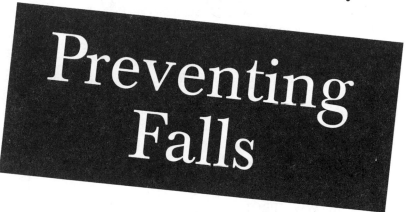

Preventing Falls

A Defensive Approach

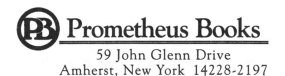

Prometheus Books

59 John Glenn Drive
Amherst, New York 14228-2197

Published 2000 by Prometheus Books

Inquiries should be addressed to
Prometheus Books
59 John Glenn Drive
Amherst, New York 14228–2197
VOICE: 716–691–0133, ext. 207
FAX: 716–564–2711
WWW.PROMETHEUSBOOKS.COM

05 04 03 02 01   6 5 4 3 2

Library of Congress Cataloging-in-Publication Data

Hutton, J. Thomas.
     Preventing falls : a defensive approach / edited by J. Thomas Hutton,
Jeffrey W. Elias, JoAnn Leavey Shroyer, and Zane Curry.
          p.   cm.
     Includes bibliographical references.
     ISBN 1–57392–761–9 (paper) – ISBN 1–57392–762–7 (video) –
ISBN 1–57392–763–6 (book & video)
     1. Falls (Accidents) in old age–Prevention. 2. Parkinson's disease–
Complications. I. Title.
RC952.5 .H87 2000
618.97–dc21   99–040082
                                                                      CIP

Printed in the United States of America on acid-free paper

Acknowledgments

The members of the Neurology Research and Education Center team wish to thank the many Parkinson's disease patients, caregivers, and families who shared their experiences, thoughts, and time in developing the Defensive Falls School.

We wish to acknowledge American Bank of Commerce and the I. Wiley Briscoe Endowment for funding that enabled us to begin the Defensive Falls School program. The support of the St. Mary of the Plains Foundation and the administration of Covenant Health System (St. Mary of the Plains Hospital) empowered us to proceed with research and education projects of the NREC providing a foundation for the development of the Defensive Falls School. We wish to thank DuPont Pharma for the grant that enabled us to produce this handbook and accompanying videotape. The illustrations on pages 66 through 78 were provided by Zane Curry, Ph.D.; the illustrations on pages 32 and 94 were provided by Trudy Hutton.

Support from all of these varied sources has made possible the development of the program and the sharing of information and suggestions to reduce the risk of falls and injuries with the Parkinson's Disease Community.

Contents

Foreword

D r. Hutton and the investigators and staff at the Neurology Research and Education Center at Covenant Health System (formerly St. Mary of the Plains Hospital) have addressed an exceedingly important aspect of Parkinson's disease: falling. Falling is an increasing problem for patients as their Parkinson's disease advances. Unfortunately, many of the causes of falling in Parkinson's disease are not amenable to drug therapy. Falling can lead to serious physical conditions and even death; therefore, the prevention of falls is an exceedingly important issue in the treatment of Parkinson's disease. Regrettably, this issue is often disregarded or not adequately addressed. The authors have provided a comprehensive program for delineating causes of falls and for preventing falls associated with Parkinson's disease and related disorders. By following such a program, Parkinson's disease patients and others can potentially prevent or at least reduce the risk of falling. While this program is called a defensive approach by the authors, it is clearly a proactive, aggressive approach to reduce falling and the fear of falling and bodily injury that results from this common symptom of Parkinson's disease. The authors clearly demonstrate an understanding of Parkinson's disease and its many motor and nonmotor symptoms essential to preventing falling in the elderly. They point out the importance of many aspects of Parkinson's disease such as vision and sensory changes that can affect balance or contribute to a fall. Importantly, they discuss many practical issues that are necessary to prevent falling and deal with freezing. By following the evaluation that the authors delineate and by executing the many defensive measures needed to make the environment safe, the parkinsonian patient will fall less.

The authors are to be congratulated on comprehensively addressing the issue of falling in Parkinson's disease which is of paramount importance, but often seriously neglected.

William C. Koller, M.D., Ph.D.
Research Director
National Parkinson's Foundation
Miami, Florida

Introduction

The risk of a serious injury from falling increases with age and represents a significant hazard to one's health and welfare. This problem is of special concern for people with Parkinson's disease. The signs and symptoms of Parkinson's disease, together with the risks attendant to advancing age, multiply the chances of falling and sustaining serious injury.

Several areas of function are important in maintaining good balance. These include

- Motor function (the ability to move about and to maneuver the body)
- Postural righting reflex (the ability to recover from a loss of balance)
- Vision
- Cognitive function (awareness, perception, and memory)

With the loss of only one of these functions, the chances remain good that the individual will maintain balance. The loss of two of these functions greatly increases the risk for falling. The loss of three or four of these functions almost guarantees a fall.

As we grow older, our eyesight begins to change. With normal daytime lighting, approximately three times more light is required to reach the retina at age sixty-five than at age twenty. With low lighting, or at night, between ten and twenty times as much light is required to reach the retina at age sixty-five as at age twenty. Memory and cognitive function may also begin to decline with age. With Parkinson's disease, motor function and postural righting reflexes are also affected.

As we age, learning to accommodate these motor, sensory, and cognitive changes is important. Any biological organism must adapt to its environment in order to thrive. In some instances, accommodations can come from within by learning new skills and coping mechanisms. In other instances, external changes are required, such as modifying the living environment or use of assistive devices.

This project represents a collaborative effort of the Neurology Research and Education Center (NREC) research investigators and staff to develop a defensive approach to reducing the risk of falling and avoiding injuries for those at risk. By teaching individuals to recognize reasons for falling and to initiate appropriate changes in their environment and lifestyles, the Defensive Falls School strives to improve quality of life and to enable the elderly to maintain mobility, independence, and dignity.

Falling Is a Major Health Risk for the Elderly

The older population of the United States is rapidly increasing. Since 1900 the number of individuals over the age of sixty-five has tripled and now represents 12.6 percent of the population. Average life expectancy has increased from 48 years in 1900 to 75.4 years in 1990. Since 1980 the rate of growth for those over sixty-five has been 24 percent while the under-sixty-five-year-old population has only grown by 9 percent. By the year 2030, those who study populations estimate that one-fifth of the population will be over the age of sixty-five. People over age eighty-five now make up about 10 percent of those over age sixty-five and in fifty years they will represent 25 percent of those over age sixty-five.

The risk of serious injury resulting from a fall increases with age. In the United States, falling is the leading cause of injuries, the fifth leading cause of death, and the second leading cause of accidental death among people over the age of sixty-five. Falling is a major cause of institutionalization and functional decline (decreasing ability to perform activities of daily living) in the senior population.

- Ten percent of falls result in serious fractures or injuries.
- Among sixty-five-year-olds, records indicate one-fourth to one-

third fall in a one year period and half of those people fall more than once.

- For those living in institutions, 10 to 25 percent have a serious fall every year.
- Twenty-five percent of these falls result in injuries that require medical attention.
- Five percent of those who fall suffer a fracture or require hospitalization; 1 percent of these injuries result in a hip fracture.
- Of those falls that result in hospitalization, approximately 50 percent of hospitalized individuals are initially discharged to nursing homes and 25 percent of these individuals continue to reside in nursing homes after one year.

Falls that occur while walking are most likely to injure the wrist or hand. Falls that occur when one is standing or transferring weight (getting up, sitting down, climbing or descending stairs, etc.), or a fall sideways or backwards, increase the risk of a hip fracture. Hip fractures are estimated to be eight times more likely to occur when one falls while turning than when one is walking straight. Women are at a greater risk for hip fractures than men due to reduced bone mass, osteoporosis, and less muscle strength.

A single cause for a fall rarely exists. Leading factors contributing to falls include created environmental hazards (e.g., stairs, change in floor height such as a ramp, or change in floor surface), gait/balance problems, muscle weakness, poor vision, inattention, and impaired judgment. Many falls can be prevented by taking deliberate preventive precautions. External environmental factors and how those factors might interact with the internal condition of the individual person must be considered. For people with Parkinson's disease and other balance disorders, falls constitute an especially real and serious problem.

Falls and Parkinson's Disease

Parkinson's disease is a slowly progressive neurological disorder that results from a loss of cells deep in the brain that produce a vital chemical called *dopamine*. The brain acts as the body's communication system by receiving stimuli from the sense organs and then transmitting the messages to various parts of the body. An interruption of the messages to the portion of the brain that controls movement may result in slow or unpredictable movement.

Parkinson's disease is primarily associated with two areas of the brain called the *substantia nigra* and the *striatum*. The striatum is the part of the brain that controls movement, posture, balance, and walking. Cells in the substantia nigra connect with the striatum and pass messages along by means of dopamine, a *neurotransmitter*, which helps the neurons in the brain communicate with each other. In Parkinson's disease, many cells in the substantia nigra, and some of the cells in the striatum, die or are damaged. As the cells degenerate, less dopamine is available. Loss of approximately 80 percent of the cells in the substantia nigra results in the appearance of Parkinson's disease symptoms: slowness, stiffness, tremor, and difficulty in balance.

The Cardinal Signs of Parkinson's disease

- Bradykinesia (slow movement)
- Tremor (rhythmic shaking; involuntary movement of part[s] of the body as a result of sequential muscle contractions)
- Rigidity or stiffness
- Loss of balance

Secondary signs of Parkinson's disease

- Walking or gait problems; decreased arm swing
- Stooped posture
- "Freezing" (a temporary, involuntary inability to move)
- Blank facial expression
- Swallowing problems
- Reduced volume in speech
- Drooling
- Mood changes
- Bowel or bladder problems

Some forms of parkinsonism can be traced to a particular cause. Certain drugs that interfere with dopamine in the brain, including some tranquilizers (e.g., haloperidol, prochlorperazine, or chlorpromizine), high blood pressure medicines, and most medicines for nausea, may cause symptoms of parkinsonism. Some patients who have suffered several small strokes may also have symptoms of parkinsonism. A virus, such as the one responsible for the encephalitis epidemic that occurred between 1918 and 1925, may cause damage to the basal ganglia, leaving people with a type of parkinsonism. The vast majority of patients, however, suffer from *idiopathic Parkinson's disease*, meaning that the cause of their disease is unknown.

A variety of scales have been developed to describe the severity of Parkinson's disease. One commonly used clinical scale was developed by Drs. Margaret Hoehn and Melvin Yahr. The Hoehn and Yahr Scale divides Parkinson's disease into five stages:

Stage I   – Signs of Parkinson's disease are unilateral, affecting only one side of the body.

Stage II   – Signs of Parkinson's disease are bilateral, but balance is not impaired.

Stage III – Signs of Parkinson's disease are bilateral and balance is affected. The person remains physically independent.

Stage IV   – Parkinson's disease is functionally disabling. The person is unable to walk or stand without some assistance.

Stage V   – The person with Parkinson's disease is confined to a bed or wheelchair.

Progression through the stages of Parkinson's disease is highly variable. In rare instances, a person may progress to stage IV or V in as little as five years. Typically, a person may have Parkinson's disease for fifteen to twenty years before entering the later stages of the disease. The staging of the disease does not take into account frequently seen clinical fluctuations resulting from the effects of medication.

The staging of an individual with Parkinson's disease is useful as a reference for predicting the risk for falling. In stages I and II there is little concern for the risk of falling. However, in stages III, IV, and V balance and mobility difficulties greatly increase the concern for the risk of falling.

In the early phases of Parkinson's disease, family members and friends may notice changes in posture, gait, and movement. These symptoms may cause or contribute to the Parkinson's disease patient's risk for falls. Thus, Parkinson's disease patients are at increased risk for falls not only because of age-related changes but also because of physiological changes that occur due to the disease.

Physiological changes contributing to increased risk of falling:

• Vision–reduced ability to see contrast
• Motor strength–reduced strength in older persons

- Coordination—rigidity, tremor, bradykinesia make previously simple movements more difficult; e.g., buttoning a shirt or eating
- Balance—reduced balance is one of the cardinal signs of Parkinson's disease
- Attention
- Executive function
- Walking speed, "freezing"—slow, shuffling steps and a sudden inability to move the feet are common

While many symptoms of Parkinson's disease can be well managed with medication, some aspects of the disease remain that are not effectively managed and that place the patient at significant risk for falling. For example, vision problems, balance, gait problems, and freezing episodes are not particularly well managed with medication and other strategies should be employed.

The Defensive Falls School

An important aspect of "successful aging" is the ability to maintain mobility and remain independent. The primary goal of
the Defensive Falls School is to make individuals aware of situations and conditions that increase the risk of falls and identify steps
they can take to limit that risk. Another goal of the Defensive Falls
School is to help participants develop confidence. Such confidence,
linked with realism, allows for continued mobility and activity.

The Defensive Falls School, as presented at the Neurology Research and Education Center, lasts approximately four hours and
includes four basic components. The school begins with a teaching
session in which the physiological causes of falls are discussed.
Included in this discussion are changes related to normal aging as
well as changes resulting from Parkinson's disease.

The second portion of the program presents practical tips and
suggestions to evaluate the home environment and lifestyle and
makes suggestions to meet current needs. During this portion of the
program, participants are encouraged to evaluate their home environments carefully, as well as their physical needs and abilities. A
major focus of the falls school program is that *one must be willing to
make changes.*

In order to reduce the risk of falling, changes may have to be made in a built environment (e.g., home, office, apartment, etc.) that is familiar and comfortable. Making changes is difficult, even with the knowledge that such changes reduce the risk of injury. Most people do not wear the same clothes or drive the same car that they did twenty years ago. They do not have the same diet or take part in the same activities that they did twenty years previously. These same people, however, frequently live in the same house with the same furniture arrangement and furnishings for many decades. As physical needs and abilities change, so must the familiar home environment.

Certain internal and external factors exist in the home environment that directly relate to the risk of falling. The internal factors are highly individual and directly related to the medical history and personal abilities of the individual with Parkinson's disease.

Internal factors directly related to the risk of falling

- Physical capability
- Mobility
- Sensory capability
- Illness
- Prescribed medications
- Cognitive ability
- General psychological state
- Fear of falling
- History of falling
- Activities of daily living
- Degree of social interaction and support

The external factors are external to the person and related to the built environment. With the factors listed below in mind, a survey of the home environment and lifestyle will empower the individual and family to recognize hazardous conditions and make the necessary changes.

External factors directly related to the risk of falling

- Floor surface and texture
- Sensory surround and feedback (auditory and visual)
- Furniture arrangement
- Structural design of furniture
- Interior lighting (quality and quantity)
- Architectural features: stairs, steps, ramps
- Wall surfaces
- Doorways

If one or more falls has already occurred, keep a journal of those falls to aid in analyzing their causes. List the location of the fall, the activity at the time of the fall, and what clothing and footwear were worn at the time of the fall. Also list physical condition and psychological state prior to the fall, medications taken, and the time of day of the fall. The understanding of what contributes to a fall is a key element in avoiding a fall.

Following the home environment session of the Defensive Falls School presentation, the NREC staff provides demonstrations for the third portion of the program. This demonstration consists of the proper methods of transfer into and out of a chair, a bed, and a car, as well as demonstrating how a caregiver can give safe assistance. The staff shows assistive devices and walking aids and discusses how and when they are best used.

The teaching portion of the Defensive Falls School is followed by individual assessment measures of seven areas of risk for falls. Once each falls school participant is assessed, he or she receives a "report card" that evaluates individual performance in each area of assessment. This evaluation gives each person an objective prediction of risk for sustaining a fall. The evaluation, coupled with the information regarding changes in the living environment and hazards in public spaces (e.g., sloping floors, clutter on floors, and steep stairways), can give the participant a proactive way to avoid falls.

Each of the individual assessments used in the Defensive Falls School contributes to the risk profile of falls school participants.

Assessment Measures for Defensive Falls School

- Fine motor coordination
- Vision
- Balance
- Gait
- Muscle coordination
- Physical examination
- Cognition

Fine Motor Coordination

Any voluntary movement of the arms or hands while in a standing position can require an adjustment of balance. Voluntary movements of the arms and hands require an anticipatory adjustment of other muscles to compensate for the direction of the force exerted by the arm or hand. An action as simple as placing a key in a lock and then pushing the door open while turning a doorknob requires several anticipatory and compensatory balance adjustments. These adjustments involve leg muscles, back muscles, and neck muscles, in addition to other muscles. The smoothness and ease of movement of the hands and arms makes anticipatory and compensatory adjustments easier and more accurate.

If frustration mounts as a result of difficulty in movement, awareness of surroundings is reduced and balance may be impaired. The task of selecting the proper key from a key ring and inserting the key in a lock changes the center of balance and challenges several functional areas.

Areas challenged by concentration on a fine motor task

- Vision
- Strength

- Attention
- Frustration
- Tolerance

Poor control of arms and hands also can lead to clumsiness with objects such as keys. This clumsiness may lead to increased frustration and loss of attention. While seemingly unrelated, the controlled use of arms and hands is important to balance and to general awareness of body motion and surroundings.

As a unit, arm and hand function can be estimated by several simple means. One that is used efficiently and effectively in the Defensive Falls School is the transfer of beans from one bowl to another bowl. A description of this assessment as a measure of the functional use of arms and hands is included in Appendix B. Longer periods of time required to complete the transfer of beans are predictive of an increased risk of a fall.

Vision and Falls in the Elderly and in Parkinson's Disease Patients

Changes in vision resulting from the normal aging process, as well as changes associated with Parkinson's disease, are significant causes of falls. The inability to see obstacles in one's path, to see changes in surface conditions, and to see dangerous situations because of stairs or ramps will increase the chances that one will fall.

AGE-RELATED CHANGES IN THE LENS OF THE EYE

Changes in vision, many noticeable by middle age, are an inevitable part of the aging process.

Basic vision changes one can expect with age

- Decreased acuity
- Decreased contrast sensitivity
- Greater sensitivity to glare
- Slower and lesser adaptation to night vision
- Decreased color vision
- Narrowed useful field of vision

Many of the changes in vision take place in the lens of the eye and represent structural changes rather than changes in central nervous system functioning. Decreased accommodation and acuity occur due to loss of flexibility in the lens and the muscles that control the lens. As one grows older, the lens in the eye becomes stiffer. The ability of the pupil to quickly respond to changes in light also diminishes. For example, the older adult may become effectively blinded temporarily when moving from a well-lit area to a poorly lit area, because the time required for the eye to make adjustments to this lighting change is increased. Accompanying this loss of flexibility in the lens is reduced visual acuity. A reduction in the widening of the pupil in dim lighting conditions permits less light into the eye. This makes details difficult to distinguish. Slowness to accommodate to light changes also gives rise to complaints of increased glare and reduced vision. Reduced lens transparency due to cataracts results in poor clarity of vision and increased susceptibility to glare. Yellowing of the lens, a normal part of aging, results in loss of perception of the blue end of the color spectrum, making the color blue more difficult to distinguish. Over a period of time, exposure to sunlight may damage the eye. Blue light waves damage the retina, while ultraviolet light from the high energy portion of the light spectrum damages the lens and encourages cataract formation. This is why sunglasses that block the blue and ultraviolet portions of the light spectrum are recommended. See Appendix B for tests for these age-related vision changes that can contribute to susceptibility to falling.

CENTRAL NERVOUS SYSTEM CHANGES AND VISION

Changes in the central nervous system due to aging also occur at the level of the retina and visual cortex. These changes bring about significant alterations in vision:

- Reduced peripheral field of vision (the outer part of the field of vision), particularly during stressful or attention-demanding situations

- Reduced visual processing speed (the time needed to search the visual field)
- Reduced speed of light and dark adaptation (the time needed to respond to changes in light)
- Loss of depth perception (the ability to perceive in three dimensions)
- Loss of ability to see contrast (the ability to distinguish details in light and dark)

GAZE

There is little change with age in the ability to maintain a steady gaze. *Dynamic* (movement-related) gaze, which involves following a moving target, however, becomes less smooth with age. Limitation of the ability to look upward may be reduced with age due to physical limitations such as arthritis of the neck, stooped posture, and drooping eyelids. Also, the ability to move the eyes upward is reduced with normal aging, and is frequently impaired or absent with Parkinson's disease. The initiation and velocity of large *saccades* (eye movements) is also reduced with normal aging. These limitations result in an increase in the time needed to study the environment to gain necessary visual information. Slower scanning of the environment means less complete visual information on which to act.

Reduced upgaze is a major indication of increased falls risk. When one must tilt the head back to look up, the center of gravity is shifted and balance is affected. The less one can look upward without moving the head, the greater the risk for a fall. Therefore, unrestricted upgaze is important in maintaining balance and avoiding a fall.

PARKINSON'S DISEASE AND VISION

Changes in vision become problems for all of us as we grow older. Parkinson's disease, however, accentuates decline in four particular

aspects beyond the expectations of normal aging. Two of these problems are related to a lack of muscle control. The ability to follow
objects in visual pursuit, such as watching movement on a television
screen, and the ability to adapt vision as one moves in one's built
environment are compromised beyond what is seen in normal aging.
This increases the possibility of a fall because of incorrect perception
of the environment (e.g., not perceiving slipperiness of a floor surface). As noted, individuals with Parkinson's disease may have
reduced ability to look up (upgaze) or down (downgaze). Research
has shown that over 90 percent of Parkinson's disease patients have
moderately to severely reduced upgaze compared to only 10 percent
of age-matched persons who do not have Parkinson's. Eye movement, rather than head movement, makes maintaining one's center
of gravity and balance easier.

The remaining two aspects of vision that show accentuated
change with the onset of Parkinson's disease involve the central nervous system. *Spatial vision* assessed by visual construction (the ability
to copy a figure), is likely to be impaired in persons with Parkinson's
disease. When asked to copy a simple line drawing, these individuals
often have difficulty reproducing how the parts should fit together.
Recognition of the objects and the correct perspective does not seem
to be impaired. The ability to copy the figures is impaired, but this
impairment does not appear to be due to loss of motor function in
arms and hands.

Research shows that visual construction and restricted upgaze are
accurate predictors of fallers and nonfallers. Using both poor visual
construction and restricted upgaze as risk factors, the Defensive Falls
School researchers were able to correctly classify 95 percent of fallers
and 63 percent of nonfallers. This can be compared to the pre-
dictability of the Unified Parkinson's Disease Rating Scale (UPDRS)
gait assessment measure that correctly classified 87 percent of fallers
and 85 percent of nonfallers. Combining the gait measures with the
visual measures allowed 100 percent accurate prediction of fallers
and 82 percent accurate prediction of nonfallers. Because falls are a
result of a combination of risk factors, a specific number or value for

an assessment does not mean a fall is impending. Nevertheless, limited upgaze and difficulty in drawing simple figures are major components of the falls school profile.

The last aspect of vision that is particularly impaired in the Parkinson's disease patient is perhaps the most important with respect to designing and living in a visual environment: The ability to perceive *contrast* in the environment becomes increasingly impaired as the disease progresses. Contrast refers to the difference in brightness between adjacent areas of a visual stimulus. For example, the doorway is more easily seen when the door frame is painted in distinct contrast to the adjacent wall. A dark door frame on a light-colored wall is a good example. Another real-life example of contrast is writing with dark ink on white paper to maximize the contrast and make the words easier to read. A person with Parkinson's disease with well corrected acuity may still have complaints that he or she "just doesn't see very well." Parkinson's disease patients frequently report vague problems with vision that glasses do not correct. The source of these complaints most likely stems from eye-movement dysfunction, loss of visual contrast sensitivity, and reduced central processing abilities.

VISUAL CONTRAST SENSITIVITY AND PARKINSON'S DISEASE

Visual contrast sensitivity involves the ability to see contrast over a range of spatial frequencies. The visual system responds to a number of visual frequencies much like a TV receives a number of frequencies that we call channels. Visual information available at high contrast (e.g., dark on light) allows the use of the high-frequency channels of the visual system. High-frequency means that there is more visual information per degree of visual angle. For example, an oil painting viewed from close range appears to be blobs of color. Standing close to the painting results in viewing the painting with a wide visual angle and perceiving it via the use of low-frequency channels. As one steps back from the painting, the visual angle is reduced and the objects can be perceived at a higher visual frequency and become recognizable. At the higher visual frequency the blobs of color become recognizable images.

High-frequency vision is superior when individuals are trying to identify objects or detect edges and boundaries between objects. The perception of dark letters on a white background requires the ability to see high spatial frequency information. Reading a note written with a sharp pencil rather than a dull pencil is easier because the sharp pencil allows the lead to be transferred to the page with greater contrast and this stimulates the high-frequency channels in the visual system. We can see the edges of steps more clearly under bright light because the light heightens the contrast and stimulates use of the high-frequency channels in the visual system.

Because people do not live in a world of constant high contrast, the use of low-frequency vision becomes important. In everyday activities, one must frequently function under low light conditions that reduce contrast. For example, when meeting a friend in a dimly lit restaurant, one must use low-frequency visual information to recognize the friend. Recognition of faces, perception of the speed of moving objects, and perception of the speed of one's own movements depend upon the ability of the visual system to respond to low frequency visual information. Although high contrast is better for detection and recognition of objects, individuals often prefer and design low contrast into everyday surroundings. High contrast is energizing; low contrast is soothing. Aesthetics should be balanced with safety concerns. Visual displays that are low contrast under high luminance become

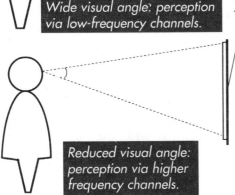

Wide visual angle: perception via low-frequency channels.

Reduced visual angle: perception via higher frequency channels.

even lower contrast under low luminance. What one views at 20/20 vision under brightly lit conditions, another may view at 20/60 vision under low light conditions, requiring the viewer to be three times closer to an object to see the same detail.

Similar to loss in normal aging, the loss of contrast sensitivity in treated Parkinson's disease patients typically begins in the high frequency channels. Eventually, contrast sensitivity is reduced in the low-frequency channels. High-frequency loss is usually detected by stage III Parkinson's and low-frequency loss becomes apparent by stage IV. This loss is well beyond that expected from normal aging. In levodopa naive Parkinson's disease patients, low-frequency loss can be detected but dopamine replacement therapy restores low-frequency vision for a time. The degree of contrast sensitivity lost varies from individual to individual. The extent of loss due to Parkinson's disease can be startling. When high-frequency visual information cannot be perceived, a component of the visual world is lost. Information not perceived cannot be processed or used in everyday functioning. What may appear to be changes in cognition and personality may be heavily influenced by changes in the ability to perceive one's surroundings. Attempts to enhance the visual environment under such circumstances may prove difficult. One must provide a high-contrast, well-lit environment.

The Built Environment and Vision

C hanges in vision result in dissatisfaction with environments. The leading complaints about built environments are:

- Environments are too dimly lit.
- Environments are too bright and produce glare.
- Environments produce changing levels of light and shadows.
- Written material is too small to read.
- Displays are too cluttered.
- Light contrast is too low to see edges and corners of objects.
- Signs are too high to be read or they arc hidden in complex displays.
- Information (lettering) on signs is too small to be read when moving.

One must analyze the environment for situations that may contribute to a fall. Low-speed transition to differing light conditions (e.g., dark to brightly lit areas or sunny spaces to dimly lit spaces) are particularly hazardous. The changes in the cornea, iris, and lens of the eye that permit less light to enter the eye cause a reduction in visual clarity and one's ability to see fine detail. Under normal lighting conditions, one-third the amount of light reaches the retina of a sixty-five-year old as reaches the retina of a twenty-year-old person. Under low light conditions, the sixty-five-year-old needs ten times the light to have the same illumination threshold as the twenty-year-old. The lower light energy colors, such as the reds, are particularly hard to see for the older individual under dim light. This makes boundaries between floor and wall surface or two floor heights particularly difficult to see when colors of the same intensity, or hue, are used. So, for example, one will have difficulty walking up stairs because he can't tell where one step ends and another begins. Lighting that produces shadows or patterns, particularly on stairs and steps, can be dangerous.

Effective visual environments are often in conflict with aesthetics, economics, and habit. Generally, conditions with more light and higher visual contrast are better if glare can be minimized. However, in the living environment, one often finds lower levels of light and reduced visual contrast, particularly at night. Lower light levels are considered more comforting, more intimate, less likely to disturb others, and less expensive than brightly lit areas. Therefore, behavior and preference for aesthetics or economics can become a risk factor for a fall. People can be short-sighted in terms of placing immediate expectations of a "pretty" environment ahead of the long-term consequences of a very expensive fall. Analyze the environment for safety first, then work with aesthetics.

Balance and Center of Gravity

Several components are required to maintain stability and balance. Balance exists when the body's center of gravity falls within the base formed by one's stance. When the center of balance moves outside this support base, a fall is more likely to occur. To maintain balance or stability, body segments must be properly aligned and changes in support surfaces must be sensed. In addition, a person must be alert to unexpected changes in balance and be able to correct for them. The degree to which this adjustment is possible will depend upon the degree to which sensory input is organized and postural strategies are effective. A number of factors in normal aging may compromise some of these aspects of balance. The person with Parkinson's disease is doubly challenged when age-related changes affecting balance are combined with changes resulting from Parkinson's disease. See Appendix B for a discussion of the balance test used by the NREC.

Age-related changes affecting balance

- Muscle weakness
- Loss of proprioception
- Changes in posture

- Orthostatic hypotension (sudden drop in blood pressure, which can lead to fainting)
- Heart arrhythmias (abnormal heart rhythm)

Medical conditions present with normal aging that may affect balance

- Combinations of medications (polypharmacy)
- Neurological disorders such as peripheral nerve damage and stroke
- Incontinence

Psychological conditions that possibly affect balance

- Changes in routine
- Changes in sleep patterns
- Fear of falling
- Resistance to change in the built environment
- Grief or depression
- Unwillingness to stay active

SENSORY ORGANIZATION AND BALANCE: PROPRIOCEPTION

Postural stability is defined as maintaining the center of body mass within specific boundaries of space, often referred to as the *limits of stability*. To maintain balance, one must maintain a proper alignment of one's center of gravity. To maintain proper alignment, one depends on feedback from sensory input. One is never completely still; even standing, the body sways slightly backward and forward. Thus, maintaining stability is a dynamic process that requires feedback from the eyes (visual), sensors in muscles and tendons in the legs and torso (proprioceptors), and the inner ear (vestibular system).

To maintain proper alignment of body segments for upright posture, one relies heavily on sensory feedback. This sensory feedback includes proprioceptive/somatosensory feedback; that is, feedback from muscles, joints, pressure and touch receptors, and visual and vestibular systems. This is a major means by which one knows that a surface is soft, uneven, tilting, or slippery. The ability to detect that a change in posture is needed is maintained reasonably well in Parkinson's disease patients. The primary difficulty for Parkinson's disease patients is in making postural corrections appropriately and efficiently. By the time one enters stage III Parkinson's disease, the righting reflex (the ability to regain balance) is impaired. Impaired righting reflexes coupled with poor muscle coordination are the major factors limiting postural corrections to balance.

When muscles work in opposition to each other, movement and somatosensory input are reduced. Stiffness or weakness in the lower extremities, particularly the ankles, results in using a hip strategy rather than ankle strategy to control sway during static (standing) balance. The strategy used is particularly relevant if floor or ground surfaces require postural adjustment. Using hip strategy, leaning forward or backward is done from the hips rather than from the ankles. Knees and ankles are kept stiff rather than flexible. When using an ankle strategy, the body rotates on an axis around the ankles. This strategy provides greater flexibility and a greater range of movement than if the body is rotated around the hips. The use of the larger muscles involved in a hip strategy is not only tiring but also limits the range of motion possible and reduces tolerance of a sudden change in posture.

Other conditions likely to contribute to poor proprioceptive feedback for balance are injuries or disease that affect ankles, knees, and hips. Most older individuals experience some arthritic problems. Other medical conditions, such as diabetes, that result in peripheral nerve damage also make changes in surface and balance less easily detected. Swelling in the feet and ankles has a similar effect.

SENSORY ORGANIZATION AND BALANCE: VISION

Visual input is important to several aspects of maintaining balance:

- Positioning the body in a vertical position relative to the ground
- Positioning and controling the motion of the head relative to the body and the surrounding environment
- Estimating speed and location of one's own body movement
- Estimating the speed of objects moving toward the body

Visual input is important for planning and anticipating motor movements. Peripheral and central vision are both important, but peripheral vision is considered more important for maintaining one's orientation, particularly when perception of movement is required. If visual input is removed, by darkness or not providing good visual cues for vertical orientation (e.g., moving in rooms or hallways with few contrasting features), the ability to maintain a center of gravity decreases, resulting in increased sway that may jeopardize stability. In the dark or in the absence of good visual cues for balance, we are forced to rely on somatosensory and vestibular input for balance. The ability to process visual input is reduced with aging and even more so with Parkinson's disease. The actual degree to which changes in vision affect balance in Parkinson's disease patients is not known. The planning and implementation of appropriate designs in the built environment to assist those with Parkinson's disease improve vertical orientation and perception of movement is important to reduce the risk of sustaining a fall.

Pronation/Supination

One of the means by which healthcare professionals assess the ability of muscles to work together is a simple clinical test (see Appendix B). The examiner asks the patient to rotate both hands back and forth at the wrist as though turning a doorknob. This movement is called pronation/supination. Slower rotation indicates a lack of flexibility and, for Parkinson's disease patients, it indicates that muscles are not working together, but are working in opposition. Fewer rotations and a reduced degree of wrist and arm rotation are predictive of an inability to correct one's posture quickly on an uneven surface. This motion of the arms and wrists is not only an indication of arm and hand use, but also reflects the degree to which muscles are able to work together.

Gait, Posture, and Risk of Falls in Parkinson's Disease

CONTROL OF GAIT

Walking is a complex task. It requires the ability to maintain control of one's posture and balance while propelling the body through space with only the feet in contact with a surface. The body's weight must be supported and momentum must be initiated, maintained, and controlled via muscular and nervous system mechanisms. The movement mechanism of walking is one of self-propulsion, so balance is constantly lost and equilibrium regained. At some point in time only one foot is on the ground and the body's center of gravity moves forward and is beyond the body until the opposite leg comes forward and the heel strikes the ground. At this point, the cycle begins again. A smooth gait requires anticipation of these shifts in balance and coordination of head, eye, trunk, arm, hip, leg, knee, ankle, and foot movements. Adaptation to changes in surface, direction, and speed of movement must be made. Self-confidence adds to the ability to complete this complex task.

AGE-RELATED CHANGES IN GAIT

One cannot state with assurance that the common changes in gait noted with age represent normal aging. Some healthcare professionals contend that changes in gait represent pathology or injury rather than result from aging. Nevertheless, expected gait changes occur with age that would take place even in the absence of Parkinson's disease. The most often noted age-related changes in gait include:

- Slower walking speed
- Shorter stride length
- Less head movement
- Wider stride
- More time supporting weight on both feet rather than one or the other (double stance phase)
- Less time moving from one foot to the other (swing phase)
- Less power at push off
- Reduced arm swing
- Reduced joint movement
- Change from heel strike to flat-foot strike

Each of these changes in gait require a greater effort to reduce demands on balance as one is moving. Similar changes in gait are noted when individuals know they are on a potentially slippery surface or are recovering physically or psychologically from a fall. Thus, some of the changes in gait with age, with injury, or with pathology could represent an attempt to compensate for lack of confidence and a fear of falling. Fear of falling has been shown to be a risk factor for falls and can alter one's gait.

GAIT AND PARKINSON'S DISEASE

The progressive decline in one's gait is a useful predictor of falls in Parkinson's disease. To reduce the risk of falls related to gait, one must consider that particular problems of gait may differ from one individual to the next. Parkinson's disease affects posture, balance during movement, propulsion, momentum, anticipation of movement, and muscle control. Studies of muscle action in Parkinson's disease patients during walking, standing, or sitting frequently report:

- Muscles tend to work continuously rather than in a cycle.
- There is a reduced level of muscle activation.
- Muscles that would normally work in alternate fashion are simultaneously activated and work against each other.

Not surprisingly, one of the more obvious changes associated with progressing Parkinson's disease is a change in gait.

ASSESSING GAIT

Gait and posture are commonly measured clinically in Parkinson's disease by use of the Unified Parkinson's Disease Rating Scale (UPDRS; see Appendix B). Although only a brief scale, this has been very helpful in predicting falls in Parkinson's disease patients. The greater the alteration of gait, the greater the risk for a fall. This assessment focuses on one's general degree of motion of arms and legs, length of steps, ability to turn, tendency to freeze, and need for assistance.

There are numerous other scales which can assess gait. Most of these scales assess gait velocity (speed); cadence (rhythm); number of steps; stride length, width, and variability of these; general posture; and motion of other parts of the body (particularly arm swing).

Parkinson's disease patients typically walk slowly and with reduced step length. As the disease progresses, the patient's gait characteristically can be described as stooped in posture and shuffling in pattern. The degree of arm movement is reduced and demonstrates a general appearance of reduced body movement. Due to reduced leg lift and flexibility, the patient's toes may drag along the floor. This is particularly likely to occur when the individual is tired.

People with Parkinson's disease have particular difficulty with initiation of movement and control of ongoing momentum. When momentum is uncontrolled, a *festinating gait* results. The individual appears to be falling forward and speeds up to compensate, resulting in short and rapid steps propelling him forward almost in a running mode. Festinating gait can occur without a stooped posture and forward weight shift, but these characteristics certainly add to the effect.

Coping with Freezing

*F*reezing is the name given to the temporary, involuntary inability to move that is fairly common among persons with advanced Parkinson's disease. One's feet may seem to stick to the floor or one may be unable to get up from a chair. The problem can occur at any time and some people are more prone to freezing episodes than others. Freezing is not responsive to any medication and requires behavioral retraining to initiate movement. The cause of this frustrating gait disturbance is unknown. Freezing creates a danger of falling because the beginning and end of a freezing episode are unpredictable. The unpredictability coupled with efforts by well-meaning companions to force the person to move may cause the person with Parkinson's disease to lose balance and fall.

Frequently, the circumstances leading to a freezing episode may be anticipated, even though a particular circumstance may not cause a freezing episode every time it is encountered. Many situations encountered in day-to-day activities lead to freezing episodes. Some of the more common situations are:

- Walking in crowds
- Walking in narrow hallways
- Being in confined spaces such as elevators or restroom stalls

47

- Sudden obstructions
- Approaching a doorway
- Over-fatigue or stressful situations

One of the ways to move smoothly through the environment is to develop a motor program. A motor program is an anticipated strategy for movement in space. Before walking down a hallway, based on experience, the kind of movements to be made are anticipated. If correctly anticipated, the attention needed for this activity is reduced. If movements in space are preprogrammed, as each movement occurs the program can be continually referred to for accuracy and the need for small adjustments. This preprograming process makes movement through space less cognitively demanding. An obstacle or unpredictable situation, such as a crowd of people, may require that the anticipated motor program end or be altered significantly, or another program developed quickly. For example, passing through a door and then reaching a stairwell requires generating another motor program.

Because freezing often occurs in situations in which an ongoing program must be altered or several programs strung together, the best suggestion for a person with Parkinson's disease is to consciously prepare for such situations. People should consider those situations that tend to cause freezing and, if possible, avoid those circumstances. Plan ahead and think about what to do to counteract freezing. There is no "official" way of getting started again and patients often develop their own unique methods of initiating movement.

Suggestions to combat "freezing"

- Stop trying to continue the activity.
- Call for help if necessary.
- Change direction: If you can't move forward, move sideways or take a step backward.
- Use a sound or rhythm to stimulate movement.
- Think of or sing a tune and then move to the beat. Marches have good rhythm.

- Count silently or out loud and then move to the count: 1-2-3, 1-2-3.
- Visualize an object, then lift your foot and try to step over the imaginary object.
- Imagine floor tiles are stepping stones and try to step from one to another.
- Use a pocket flashlight to throw a pool of light in front of you; try stepping in the pool.
- If you use a cane, draw an imaginary line on the floor and try stepping over the line.
- Ask a companion to place a handkerchief or piece of paper on the floor; try to step over the object.
- If you tend to freeze in a specific place, such as a doorway, try to visualize beyond the obstacle. Once beyond the object, freezing will not likely occur.

High-Risk Conditions and Built Environment Interventions

Tripping is arguably the most common reason for a fall. Parkinson's disease patients are at particular risk for a trip due to their shuffling gait in which the foot is not lifted high enough off the surface. This creates a tendency for a toe to drag or catch. This condition shifts the center of balance forward, requiring corrective action and an immediate restoration of center of gravity closer to the body. Because of rigidity of muscles, reduced stride length, and slow gait in Parkinson's disease, even small shifts forward can result in a need for correction. Correction and return to center of balance is hindered by muscle stiffness or rigidity, slowness of movement, and difficulty in generating the momentum needed to bring the tripping or alternate foot forward to regain balance. Walking with a flat-foot strike or toe strike (toe first), rather than a heel strike (heel first), is more likely to add to the difficulties caused by a shuffling gait if the surface walked on is likely to catch the foot rather than let it slide. Thick pile carpet, grass, and rough stone walkways are examples of such surfaces.

SURFACE TRANSITION AREAS

The surface walked on and footwear worn take on added importance for individuals who can't step up very high, those who drag their feet, or those who have a shuffling gait. Many homes have several different kinds of floor surface areas that require different step height, stride length, and walking speed. Common surfaces found in the home include thick or long-pile carpet, thick tile, wood, and stone floors. Transition from one surface to another requires a change of motor program. Surfaces may require a need for a change from a flat-foot strike to a heel strike or vice versa. With an unimpaired gait, many of these alterations are done easily and automatically. With an impaired gait, the alterations require a more conscious effort. Because of reduced automatic movements, people with Parkinson's disease must be especially wary of surface changes when they walk.

For individuals with impaired gait, transition points in surface friction can be particularly troublesome due to difficulty in changing motor programs necessary to adapt to the different surfaces. These transitions are even more troublesome when vision problems exist and poor lighting conditions reduce the ability to perceive and anticipate the surface change. A feeling of familiarity in the environment often makes one less conscious of changes in surfaces. For example, walking from tile to carpet requires an increase in foot height clearance.

Quite often, transitions in surface are accompanied by transitions in light, elevation, visual, and auditory complexity. An area that provides good visibility in bright lighting or in the daytime may have poor visibility at night. In familiar settings a person tends to adapt gait based on long experience with the necessary gait changes. In unfamiliar places such transition areas can be especially dangerous if the individual does not make a conscious effort to be aware of necessary changes.

Footwear can play an important role as well. Rubber- or crepe-soled shoes may be good for traction and support on tile, but may catch on a high-pile rug or a rougher surface. Unlike automobile tires, no one has developed a shoe that can perform well on all surfaces.

Stepbacks, Turn Areas, Acceleration Zones, and Elevation Changes

Turning is a high-risk factor for a fall. Turning-related falls often result in hip fracture. Spaces where stepping backward or turning in a tight space is common should be examined for ease of foot clearance and for objects that one may back into or fall over. These areas include doors that open inward; cupboards, closets, or space near frequently used appliances; bathroom or wall mirrors; and telephones on walls or on side tables. The foot should not catch on a rug or other surface during the turn. One should have a clear path once the turn is completed. Placing a mirror or picture to be examined on a wall near or opposite a low-lying piece of furniture, such as a coffee table, can be particularly hazardous because of the distraction it creates. Area rugs or carpet runners are frequently placed on top of carpet in places where there is prolonged standing or heavy traffic. This is a deadly combination when gait consists of low stepping height.

Entrances to major highways often have acceleration lanes. Homes, offices, and public areas also have acceleration zones. These are areas where gait is likely to be accelerated. We frequently move quickly to the telephone, door, home alarm system control pad, or sometimes to the bathroom, as a matter of habit. Likely acceleration areas should be examined for foot clearance and obstacles in the pathway. Areas around chairs, sofas, and beds are frequently used to gain momentum and should be examined for stability and safety.

While this kind of detective work may seem a tedious exercise in the home, the assessment is well worth the time when one considers the increased risk for a fall by elderly individuals or Parkinson's disease patients. When conducting these environmental assessments, remember that vision might be impaired and that changing lighting conditions at different times of the day may impair perception. What seems safe to a person with good vision and gait is often not safe for the person with poor vision and gait. Vision, gait, and balance deficits must be kept in mind as the home environment is assessed.

SLIPS, SLIDES, AND SLUMPS

Changes in elevation of the walking surface are not only a frequent cause of stumbling, but are often the source of slips, slides, and slumps or collapse. Stairs are a fairly obvious source of such problems. Most people with gait or balance difficulties are cautious about stairs and take proper precautions. However, bad habits sometimes take precedence over precaution. Objects to be carried up or down stairs are often placed on the steps. Carrying objects, particularly in front of the body, makes recovering from loss of balance difficult, and pushes the body's center of balance forward. Reading or turning the head to talk to others while walking up and down stairs provides a good reason to have the number of a good ambulance service handy. Stairs should certainly not be turn areas or acceleration zones. Securely attached handrails on stairs are particularly important for initiation and control of momentum. Handrails are also useful in hallways.

Stairs should be well lit at all times of day and night and not subject to glare. One should not be required to alter the center of balance to reach a light switch. Light switches should be easily accessible and installed at both the top and bottom of the stairway. Each step should be clearly distinguishable and be at an expected height. The top and bottom step should not be unexpectedly different in elevation from the other steps.

Single steps are often more dangerous than a stairway. Moreover, single steps rarely have handrails. Single steps up and down are dangerous not only because they, like stairs, require a change in motor program, but also because they do not elicit the same level of caution. Steps are often found in transition areas such as

- House to walkway
- House to porch
- Porch to yard
- Entryway to living room
- Kitchen to family room

The very location of these steps compounds their danger. Occasionally, single steps are found in acceleration areas and in backup and turn areas. These single steps deserve the same respect as a series of steps. The same precautions should be used.

Impaired gait in those with Parkinson's disease increases the risk for falling, for a variety of reasons: difficulties in initiating or controlling momentum, changing gait quickly, or changing a motor program. Design hazards in the home as well as in public areas compound the risk of falls. A suggested means to reduce the risk for falling is to be especially aware of those areas that are likely to increase risk—such as transition areas including elevation as well as surface changes, turn areas, and acceleration areas—and make a conscious effort to adjust gait accordingly.

In one's home as well as in public buildings, the *built environment,* one must be aware of *fall zones*—those areas in which one has either fallen in the past or in which the situation or circumstances are such that the built environment will likely contribute to a trip, a stumble, or a fall. Common fall zones include areas with a single step, areas congested with low furniture (e.g., foot stool or coffee table), and areas where the floor surface suddenly becomes smooth (e.g., kitchen or bathroom). These problem areas and circumstances are magnified at night or in unfamiliar areas.

Executive Function and Falls in Parkinson's Disease

Parkinson's disease affects not only motor function, but sensory functioning and cognitive processes as well. Behavior changes associated with Parkinson's disease include depression and motivation, speech and language difficulties, memory, attention, and most importantly, executive function. With respect to falling and the built environment, the changes in behavior most important to people with Parkinson's disease are those involving executive function.

BEHAVIOR AND EXECUTIVE FUNCTION

Executive function involves selecting, inhibiting, organizing, sequencing, monitoring, motivating, and mentoring aspects of behavior. Any environment constantly presents a number of stimuli to which one can respond. We *select* the stimuli we wish to respond to and *inhibit* or ignore the others. To execute a plan of behavior it must be *organized* and carried out in the appropriate *sequence* while remembering what has been done and what must still be done. To carry out this sequence, particularly if the task is new, we have to *monitor* ongoing behavior and retain *motivation* to stay on task and avoid being disturbed. Intruding thoughts, behavior, or stimuli have to be

57

inhibited. Frequently shifting back and forth between several tasks or monitoring one task while doing another is required. If we are interrupted in carrying out a task, we need to be able to focus and return to the original task. Over a period of time we need to have insight into our general behavior and evaluate our success. This latter process involves serving as a *mentor* for ourselves.

ATTENTION AND EXECUTIVE FUNCTION

In addition to selecting and executing a plan of action, executive function involves generating, focusing, and maintaining attention. Maintaining attention is crucial to having a good memory. Susceptibility to distraction is a characteristic of people who are too busy, depressed, overworked, tired, or showing signs of neurological impairment. Susceptibility to distraction increases with normal aging. Without knowing all these conditions, it is hard to tell if a person's susceptibility to distraction represents neurological impairment or life circumstances. Life circumstances can certainly contribute to the increased distractibility often seen with neurological disorders.

PROGRESSION OF EXECUTIVE FUNCTION DECLINE

Decline in executive function and the ensuing problems of distraction, motivation, and attention are the most obvious changes in cognition associated with Parkinson's disease. A brief, fifteen-minute interview called the Executive Function Test (EXIT) is a good tool to quickly assess executive function (see Appendix B). Research shows that by the time one reaches stage III Parkinson's disease approximately half of those individuals tested have executive function deficits that interfere with daily functioning. Most individuals at stage IV Parkinson's disease show executive function difficulties.

Another frequently used quick test of cognitive function that focuses on memory, language, and orientation is the Mini-Mental

State Exam (MMSE; see Appendix B). In the early stages of executive function decline, the EXIT is a good predictor of functional activities and the MMSE is not.

EXECUTIVE FUNCTION AND FALLS

A decline in executive function leads to susceptibility to falls for several reasons. Distraction in any setting is a dangerous situation relative to falls. Most accidents occur because of inattention or lack of thinking ahead. The difficulties with gait and balance in Parkinson's disease compete for attention even without executive function impairment. With executive function impairment, maintaining attention to balance and gait, as well as monitoring the environment, becomes more of a challenge. Added to this problem are changes in vision that make elements within the built environment less visable and more confusing.

The term "environmental dependency" is often used to describe how a particular aspect of the environment can seize attention and pull it away from an ongoing event. For example, when the doorbell rings the sound has such prominence that we rush to answer the door without thinking about falling. The path to the front door is often an acceleration area that has a history of slips and trips. The example of the doorbell is described as having "frontal pull." The ringing doorbell is so compelling and response so automatic that attention is pulled toward the sound and away from such hazards as an area rug or a wet floor. Turning off house security alarms or answering a telephone are other events that can grab attention and increase the risk for a fall.

In a familiar environment one can sometimes function almost without needing executive skills. The events of the day and the familiarity of the surroundings and routine pull us along. Sometimes, individuals with declining executive skills can survive reasonably well in a familiar environment and regular routine. If the environment changes, however, the change brings on a decline in self-motivation, an inability to inhibit responses to competing stimuli, and an inability to organize coherent responses in the new environment. The greater the environmental "press" of stimuli, the less coherent the individual's behavior is likely to be.

Often, individuals can function quite well when events follow a familiar course. Human information processing systems are designed to be efficient. However, when events change, new behavior patterns must be developed. Driving in a familiar neighborhood to a familiar store with familiar displays and familiar people might be done quite well in spite of declining executive function. If the car breaks down or one is involved in an accident, the new situation can disrupt the task of driving home to the point where no new competent plan can be developed. Without a familiar pattern the individual may appear to be lost or disoriented and may revert to previous behavior patterns. When one is confused, using old patterns of behavior is easier than generating new behaviors. Upon return to a familiar environment and routine, executive functioning appears competent again. These kinds of situations need to be anticipated if the stage III or IV Parkinson's disease patient lives alone or must fend for himself or herself for several days without the aid of someone else's executive function.

Anticipating Falls and Reducing Distractions

In the event of declining executive impairment, the familiar can be both friend and foe. Familiar environmental events that evoke unwanted "environmental pull," such as doorbells, alarms, and telephones, can be anticipated and modified appropriately; for example, reducing the volume of doorbells, carrying a portable telephone, or using an intercom. The establishment of routines, planning out the day ahead of time, and elimination of distractions can be very helpful. Repeating needed information verbally, by note, by computer, or by calendar helps keep plans organized. The rearrangement of environments and the change of routines should be done with executive function in mind. Last, but not least, if information is not seen or heard, it is not useful. Often, changes in vision or hearing, rather than poor memory or executive function, are the causes of poor performance.

Physical Evaluation

D uring the physical evaluation in the Defensive Falls School, the Parkinson's disease patient is assessed for additional physical risk factors that can contribute to falls. Physical assessments include medication history, blood pressure measurement, cognitive function, and completion of a modified Unified Parkinson's Disease Rating Scale. Results of the physical evaluation are recorded on the "Parkinson's Disease Fall Profile" (see Appendix C). The Parkinson's Disease Fall Profile is a tool developed by the research staff at the Neurology Research and Education Center to record results obtained from various assessments completed during the Defensive Falls School.

A complete medication history is obtained for each patient. The completed medication history may reveal additional risk factors for falls because some medications, or the inappropriate combination of several medications, can produce side effects such as light-headedness, dizziness, and confusion. Being aware of possible effects of medication allows the patient to take special precautions to avoid additional risks for falls and injury.

Blood pressure is measured to assess for orthostatic hypotension, which is frequently seen in Parkinson's disease. This sudden drop in blood pressure due to a change of position can be a direct result of

Parkinson's disease, or a side effect of medications. With this rapid decrease in blood pressure, the patient can feel light-headed and dizzy. An extreme consequence in this situation would be a fainting episode that could result in serious injury to the patient.

Mental status testing is completed during the physical evaluation to assess cognitive function. The Folstein Mini-Mental State Examination (MMSE) is administered to assess orientation, registration, attention, calculation, recent recall, comprehension, reading and writing, and the ability to draw or copy figures.

The Unified Parkinson's Disease Rating Scale (UPDRS) is a standardized assessment for determining the severity of Parkinson's disease. Only certain parts of the UPDRS are beneficial in predicting falls; therefore, a modified version is used in the falls school. It includes assessment of the following:

- Fall history
- Freezing
- Gait
- Posture
- Balance
- Bradykinesia
- Rigidity
- Resting tremor

After the assessment is completed, the patient is staged using the Hoehn and Yahr scale to assess severity of the Parkinson's disease and potential for increased risk of falls.

Home Safety Assessments

An individual with Parkinson's disease has an increased risk of an injurious fall due to the physical attributes of the disease. In addition, the built environment is fraught with hazardous conditions for the individual with Parkinson's disease. The first step to a safer living environment is to recognize that changes in one's physical condition strongly indicate that changes should be made in the environment to reduce the risk of a fall. Individuals must be willing to change the physical environment and to recognize that some items, furniture arrangements, and architectural features are no longer safe and do not promote the health and welfare of the individual with Parkinson's disease.

One should be proactive when it comes to risk of falling. Assess the environment and make the necessary changes before a fall occurs. We encourage you to make changes that will assist you or your loved one in living a comfortable, healthier, and safer lifestyle. The information that follows can serve as a checklist to use in evaluating the living environment for safety.

BATHROOMS

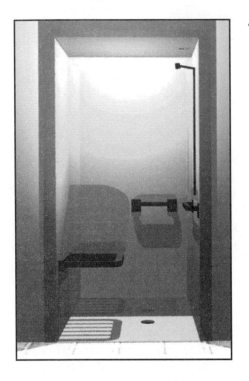

• Shower stalls should be equipped with benches, handrails, and a handheld shower nozzle. These features are easy to use and reduce the risk of a fall in the shower. This area is considered a high-risk environment and you need to take every precaution for your safety.

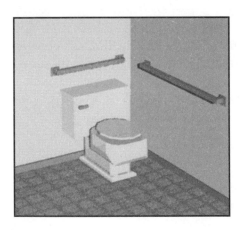

• Grab-bars should be professionally installed at appropriate heights, angles, and locations for maximum safety and security for the user.
• Examine the handrails. Different styles and designs are available for you to choose from at your local retail stores. Select the style and design that best suits your needs.
• A nonskid mat in front of the toilet is beneficial to maintain foot position as you sit and stand.

- Adhesive-backed appliques for bottoms of tubs and showers are easily installed and provide slip resistance to the floor surface.
- Use nonskid mats in tubs or showers. These mats can be laundered and can be found in different sizes to fit most tubs and showers.
- If floor-surface slipperiness is a problem, place nonskid mats outside of the tub or shower to step onto and to maintain foot placement.

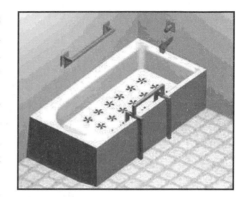

- Have grab-bars professionally installed on walls around the tub at comfortable heights, angles, and locations for your maximum safety and security.
- Be sure you can comfortably grip the bars. Many different styles and designs are available for you to purchase. Select the style and design that is best for you.

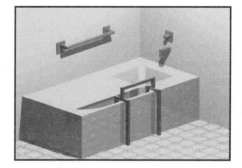

BEDROOMS

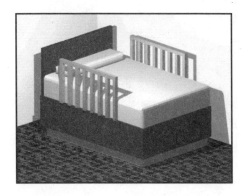

- Install side rails on both sides of your bed to increase safety and aid you in getting into the bed and getting out of the bed as well as for repositioning during sleep.
- When rising, sit on the side of the bed for a few moments before standing and walking. This pause can reduce the risk of dizziness and possibly losing your balance, resulting in a fall.

KITCHENS

You should consider the following suggestions to reduce the need for bending and stretching that can lead to a loss of balance resulting in an injurious fall.

- Arrange items in kitchen cabinets according to frequency of use, at a height that is right for you.
- Install sliding pull-out kitchen shelves in lower cabinets for easier accessibility of frequently used items.
- Use a "reacher" when possible for infrequently used items in kitchen cabinets.
- Install lazy-susans or use portable lazy-susans that can assist you in reaching items in kitchen cabinets.

LIVING AREAS

- Avoid highly polished floor surfaces that reflect mirror-like images. Many floor finish products are available in the marketplace that provide you the shine of a high polish yet are slip resistant.
- Incidents of freezing episodes have been reported that were caused by the mirrorlike images. Consider using a lower-gloss floor finish.

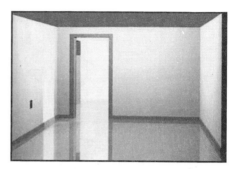

- Notice the rug on the floor between the chair and sofa. The turned-up corner is extremely hazardous and a major risk factor that can lead to a fall. If you fall in this area, you will likely hit a piece of furniture. The rug should be removed or its corners adhered to the floor surface to reduce the risk of a fall.

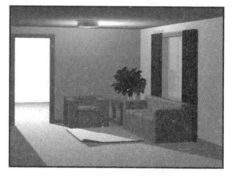

- Telephone cords or electrical cords should never be in heavy traffic areas.
- Consider alternatives in furniture placement that might eliminate the use of telephone or electrical cords.

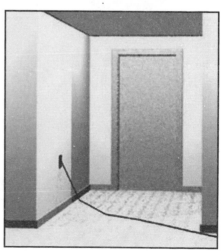

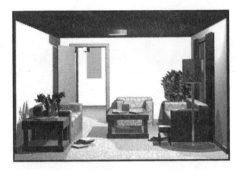

- To reduce the risk of a fall, remove all magazines, books, newspapers, and other items from the floor around your seating areas. This is considered a major risk factor that can result in a fall.
- Do you really need a coffee table? Consider removing this item of furniture from your home. Coffee tables restrict traffic patterns and reduce usable space.
- You should be able to walk across a room without having to walk around clutter on the floor. Pay careful attention to low-lying objects such as coffee tables, foot stools, sewing supplies, pets, and children on the floor. If possible, remove the clutter.

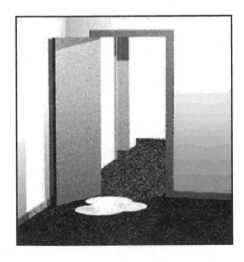

- Spilled liquids should be mopped up as quickly as possible. Do not plan to come back later to clean up the spill—you may forget.
- Use a sponge mop or sponge wipes for fast and maximum absorbency. Thoroughly dry the area after mopping.

- Pay careful attention to floor surface changes (hard to soft; soft to hard; smooth to rough; rough to smooth). This change may require adjustment in gait, posture, and balance.
- Stooped posture, unsteadiness, balance problems, and a reduction in the natural arm swing when walking make your undivided attention to floor surface changes particularly important to your safety.
- Carpet with short, dense pile is recommended. This decision is particularly important if you are experiencing problems with mobility, balance, and unsteadiness.

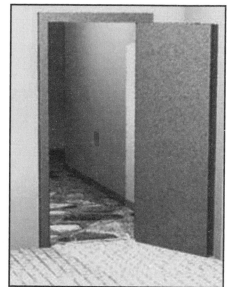

- Dimmer switches should be installed at both ends of hallways and corridors for ease in adjusting light for visual clarity. Also, consider a glow-in-the-dark switch that can be seen in dimly lit areas.
- Have lighting continuously turned on during the evening and night hours.
- Remove obstructions from hallways, such as small tables and benches that you can stumble or trip over.
- Rugs, if used, should be securely fastened to the floor to increase your sefety and minimize your risk of a fall.

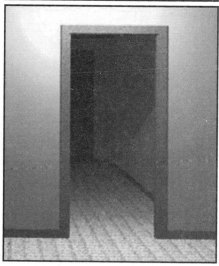

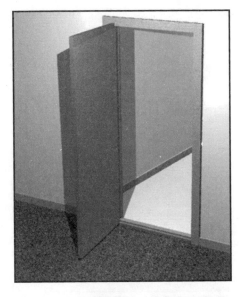

• Thresholds, if raised, should be clearly defined to draw your attention to the surface change. Your foot must be raised to safely step over the threshold. A piece of contrasting colored tape along the threshold easily marks this change. Never step on the threshold; this can affect balance.
• When possible, interior thresholds should be flush with the floor surface.

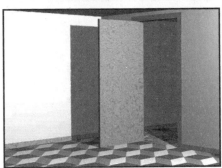

• When selecting floor coverings, be sure to examine the repeat patterns. Avoid busy repeat patterns that create optical illusions that seriously affect your depth perception.
• Small sample squares of floor covering are not large enough to provide you with a true picture of how your floor will look when installation is complete. Ask your vendor to provide a larger sample or a picture of the covering laid on a large area.

AREA RUGS

- Avoid the use of area rugs or floor cloths as much as possible. Area rugs are considered to be a major contributor to the risk of falls, trips, and stumbles.
- Select rugs and floor cloths with slip-resistant backing.
- Apply antislip tape to edges of rugs to bond the rug to the floor. This tape will keep rugs and cloths in place and flat on the floor.

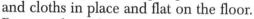

- Be sure edges of area rugs or floor cloths are securely fastened to the floor for maximum slip resistance and to keep the rug wrinkle free.
- Examine rugs periodically for tears, ravels, and deterioration, to see if repairs are needed.

CHAIRS

- One chair size and design does not fit all. When you are selecting a chair, consider the purpose of the chair (dining, relaxing), your physical attributes (height, weight), and location of the chair in the living environment (carpeted floor surface, hard floor surface).
- If you sit in an inappropriately designed chair that places pressure on the buttocks and thighs, blood circulation to the lower extremities (legs and feet) can be restricted. The restricted blood flow leads to swelling, cramping, or numbness in the legs and feet that can contribute to an injurious fall when rising from the chair and then walking.
- Select a chair that allows your feet to rest firmly on the floor when you are seated. This permits your weight to be equally distributed and provides for good balance when rising and sitting. Avoid overstuffed chairs or recliners, which may be hard to get into and out of.

- Armrests should be of a width and height that suits your body size. Both of your arms should fit comfortably on both armrests at the same time. You should not be required to lean to one side of the chair or the other to use the armrests. The armrests should be at a height comfortable for you when your shoulders are relaxed.
- The chair backrest should extend to your shoulder blades and be contoured to give you comfortable fit and provide adequate support for your upper back.

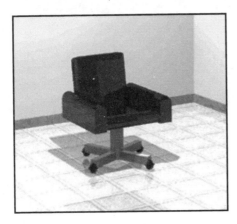

- Chairs on rollers/casters are hazardous if located on hard floor surfaces. When you are sitting down or rising, casters can roll uncontrollably and cause you to lose your balance and fall.

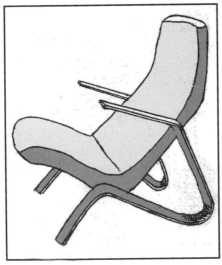

- This chair seat design tilts back, making it difficult to push your body to a standing position.

• Chairs of this design are unstable because they are lightweight and can easily be
tipped over, resulting in an
injurious fall.

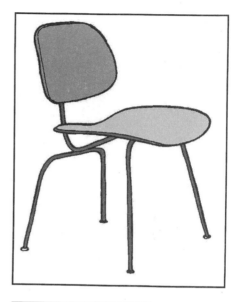

• This chair design is stable and
has curved armrests for a firm
grasp when sitting down and
rising.

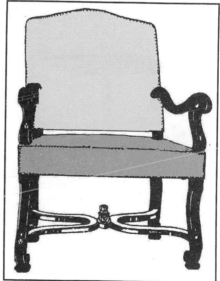

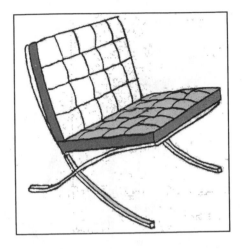

• A chair without arms does not support your weight when you are rising or sitting.

TABLES

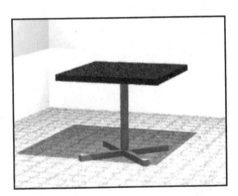

• Tables with pedestal bases should not be used to support your weight when sitting or rising. Tables of this type may be unstable and can easily be tipped over, resulting in an injurious fall.

STAIRS

- Light switches should be placed at a convenient height at both the top and bottom of stairs.
- Stair rails should be installed on both sides of stairs at the appropriate height for your maximum safety.
- Riser and tread surface can be varied in color or pattern for visual clarity.
- Antislip tape with reflective or glow-in-the-dark stripes can be applied to the edge of each step inexpensively and easily for safety. This tape is excellent for exerior steps to assure good visibility.

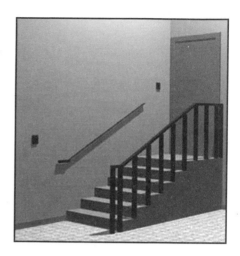

- Stair rails should be installed on both sides of stairs at an appropriate height for maximum safety.
- Mirrors used as the bottom riser can be confusing and create optical illusion.
- Stairs should have the horizontal edge of each step clearly marked to avoid missing a step.

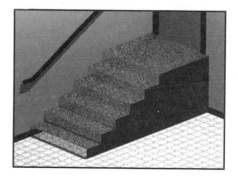

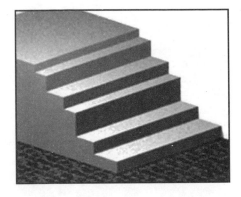

- Before walking up or down stairs, take time to observe the risen height and tread depth. Sometimes these factors are not equal for each step, which can create a serious hazard.
- All stairs should be well lit during all hours of the day and night for your safety and welfare.
- Most falls on stairs occur while descending, so you should pay special attention when going down stairs.

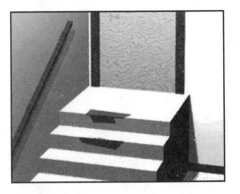

- You should repair or replace torn or frayed surfaces on stairs as soon as you notice the problem. The illustration to the left portrays a serious hazard.
- Loose stair surfaces should be fastened securely to avoid a slip resulting in an injurious fall.

Note: Stairs should have firmly attached handrails on both sides. The handrails in the drawing above have been omitted for illustration purposes only.

Transfer Techniques

With the limitations in flexibility, mobility, and strength experienced by many Parkinson's disease patients, effective techniques for repositioning and maneuvering through the environment are essential. The use of proper transfer techniques can increase the patient's level of independence by decreasing the need for assistance from others. An additional benefit is reduced incidence of falls and injury, not only to the patient, but also to the caregiver.

The Parkinson's disease patient experiences special difficulty when getting into and out of a chair, a bed, or a car because these actions produce a shift in the body's center of gravity. Special care must be taken to avoid losing one's balance and falling. When using any of the following transfer methods, break the action into its separate parts and think carefully about each step as it is performed. Concentrating on the motion makes one more aware of the shifts in balance and reduces the likelihood of a fall.

Tips for sitting in a chair

- Approach the chair as closely as possible.
- Turn so that your back is to the chair.
- Back up carefully until you feel the chair against your legs.
- To sit down, bend forward slightly and lower the body into the chair.
- Use arms of the chair when possible for balance and guidance.

Tips for getting out of a chair

- Place feet slightly apart, partially under the front of the chair.
- Slide forward until you are sitting on the front edge of the chair.
- Place your hands on the chair armrests.
- Bend forward so that your nose is over your knees.
- Push on armrests and boost up, leaning forward until you are on your feet.
- Rocking back and forth several times may help boost you up more easily.

Tips for getting out of bed

- Lie on your back.
- Bend your knees up, placing your feet flat on the bed.
- Turn on your side, reaching your arm across your body to assist rolling over.
- Scoot to the edge of the bed, alternating moving the shoulders, then the hips, a little at a time.
- Slide your feet off the edge of the bed.
- Use your arms to push yourself into a sitting position ("walk" your hands to help you push into a sitting position).
- A side rail or chair fastened to the side of the bed may be helpful.
- Once you are in a sitting position, stay there several seconds, making sure you are not dizzy.

- Follow the directions to get out of a chair. Push on the bed with your hands if you do not have a side rail or a sturdy piece of furniture to push up on.

Tips for getting into bed and lying down

- Following the previous instructions for sitting in a chair, sit on the edge of the bed.
- Lift legs onto the bed (one at a time may be easier).
- Using arms for support, lower yourself into lying position.
- Slide to center of bed, moving hips, then shoulders until you are in a comfortable position.

Tips for getting into a car

- Be sure the car is parked far enough away from the curb so that you can step onto level ground before getting in or out of the car. Approximately twelve inches from the curb is recommended.
- Turn so that you are backing into the car for the last steps.
- Follow suggestions for sitting in a chair.
- Sit on the seat so that your buttocks lead.
- Sit down on the seat, then swing your legs into the car.
- Slide over in the seat so that you are comfortably positioned in the car.
- A plastic bag or satin seat cover placed on the seat will make sliding easier.
- You can have a handle attached to the dashboard or door frame by an auto body shop to make getting in and out of the car easier.

Tips for getting out of a car

- Slide to the edge of the seat.
- Swing both legs out of the car.

- Place feet slightly apart, centered in front of you.
- Lean forward and stand up as for rising from a chair.
- Avoid putting weight on door frame, which may be unsteady; hold on to the body of the car for balance if necessary.

Dizziness:
Orthostatic Hypotension

Many patients with Parkinson's disease experience a drop in their blood pressure when changing from a lying or sitting position to a standing position. The medical term for this is *orthostatic hypotension*. While orthostatic hypotension is experienced in normal aging, it may also be a side effect of antiparkinson medication. This is not unusual because many of the antiparkinson medications tend to lower one's blood pressure. One of the dangers associated with orthostatic hypotension is loss of balance leading to a fall.

The most common symptom of orthostatic hypotension is lightheadedness or dizziness, with or without feeling faint. Weakness and loss of consciousness can occur if the drop in blood pressure is severe. If dizziness or lightheadedness occurs when changing from a sitting or standing position, the following suggestions may be helpful. Consult your physician about the suggestions that might be helpful to you.

Tips to combat orthostatic hypotension: dizziness or lightheadedness

- Sit on the edge of the bed or chair for a few minutes before getting up.
- Exercise your feet and legs prior to rising from the bed or a chair.

83

- Stand up slowly, holding a sturdy piece of furniture or a walker.
- Keep the head of your bed tilted upward at a 30° angle, either using an electric bed or blocks placed under legs at the head of the bed.
- Consult your physician about adding salt to your food to help maintain blood pressure.
- Drink a cup of regular coffee after meals to maintain blood pressure.
- Eat small, frequent meals (four to six per day).
- Sit down after exercise to prevent pooling of blood in the feet.
- Wear elasticized stockings (thigh-high are recommended) to promote blood flow from your feet and legs.

If these measures fail, a change in antiparkinson medications or the addition of another medication to aid in maintaining blood pressure may be necessary. Discuss your options with your physician.

Walking Aids and Assistive Devices

Walking aids and other assistive devices need to be considered if falls are occurring as a result of balance or gait problems that cannot be corrected by changes in the physical environment, medication, or behavior retraining. The most secure ambulatory device is a walker. For ease of use and safety, a walker with locking wheels that engage when weight is applied to the walker is recommended. This type of walker is easy to move and gives maximum security for stopping. A basket or bag can be attached to the front of the walker that is useful for carrying items. Other types of walkers are lightweight and aluminum framed, either with or without wheels. These walkers may not be as helpful if the user tends to fall backward because they are lightweight and may fall on top of the user, rather than providing support for balance.

The use of a walking stick or hiking stick may lend support and aid in balance. The height of such a stick encourages the user to stand straighter and maintain center of gravity. A cane may be difficult to use for a person with Parkinson's disease due to decreased natural arm swing. The low height of the cane encourages leaning forward, a dangerous position for people whose stooped posture already tends to cause the center of gravity to be shifted forward.

A transfer belt is an inexpensive device to assist a person in rising from a sitting position. To use this device, place the belt around the patient's waist or chest. Ask the patient to follow the steps for getting out of a chair. The caregiver should position himself or herself in front of the patient with knees against the patient's knees. The caregiver bends his or her knees slightly and firmly grasps the belt on each side of the patient. As the patient pushes on the armrests of the chair to stand up, the caregiver pulls upward on the belt. Both patient and caregiver will stand together. The caregiver must remember to use his legs to help pull upward; to avoid the risk of back strain, do not let the back do the work.

For persons who are unsure of their balance or have had numerous falls, a wheelchair or electric "scooter" is recommended, especially when in public and away from the familiar home environment. Another assistive device to aid balance is the long-handled "reacher." This device allows one to reach items on very high shelves or to pick up objects off the floor without having to lean over or squat down.

Recovery from a Fall

If a fall does occur, there are steps one can take to recover. Because falling is a very real danger for the older population and for individuals with Parkinson's disease, in particular, practicing a recovery strategy is a good idea. Consider having someone on hand who can assist you in case you have trouble getting up, even from this practice session. Lie on the floor, pretending you have fallen, and follow these steps.

- Remain still for a few moments to calm yourself.
- Move your arms and legs slowly to see if there is any injury. If there is any extreme pain at any site, take care not to injure the site further.
- Turn on your side and push up to a sitting position by "walking" your hands up to your waist while pushing your body up.
- Sit in this position a moment or two, again checking for injury.
- Turn over to your hands and knees and crawl to a sturdy chair.
- Position hands on each side of the chair seat.
- Bend the stronger leg at the knee and put your foot flat on the floor. Push up to a standing position.
- Turn around slowly and sit on the chair.

- If you are unable to get up by yourself using the chair, crawl to a telephone and call for help.
- If you are unable to crawl, try scooting on your back or side to a telephone.

Conclusion

The topic of preventing falls is especially important for persons with Parkinson's disease. The Neurology Research and Education Center staff became interested in falls prevention because of falls reported by both patients and their caregivers. These reports included hip fractures and other injuries. Hip fractures in the older population result in substantial injury, and even death. Of falls that result in hospitalization, 50 percent of the patients are discharged to a nursing home. Twenty-five percent of those patients will still be in the nursing home after one year. Reports also included environmental factors that contributed to falls and resulted in injuries. These incidents make falling a major cause of institutionalization and resulting functional decline.

The ability to move and remain independent are intertwined. Even if no injury results, a fall can cause a person who has functioned independently to limit activity because of the fear of falling again and sustaining an injury. This reduction in activity can lead to a downward spiral of inactivity, including loss of exercise and reduced social and mental stimulation. Such loss can lead to decreased functioning in the person's home, thus setting the stage for another fall.

Keeping a person active, mobile, and as independent as possible is of utmost importance. A fall seldom "just happens"; many falls can be prevented. A number of preventive measures presented in this handbook and the accompanying videotape can be utilized in the home and in public places to reduce the risk of falling. The price of a little prevention represents a major health bargain for the individual with Parkinson's disease.

Our goal for the Defensive Falls School is to promote personal dignity, safer mobility, and functional independence of the person with Parkinson's disease and for others susceptible to falls. The Defensive Falls School presentation provides information that can reduce the risk of a fall in the home and in public places. The key element to preventing falls in the built environment is the *willingness to change the environment*!

Appendix A

Defensive Falls School Curriculum

The Neurology Research and Education Center has developed a model curriculum for a Defensive Falls School. The information in the handbook offers a synopsis of the material presented to Defensive Falls School participants. Participants are also given a variety of printed material on the risk factors for falls and suggestions for avoiding falls. The schedule for the Defensive Falls School found to be the most effective is as follows:

- Overview and Introduction of Falls School Staff
- Lecture: Physiological Factors Contributing to Falls
- Question and Answer Session; Participant Comments
- Lecture: Environmental Factors Contributing to Falls
- Question and Answer Session; Participant Comments
- Break; Refreshments
- Individual Assessments
- Individual Evaluations
- Final Questions and Comments

The staff of the Neurology Research and Education Center Defensive Falls School suggests that the number of participants in a Defensive Falls School be small to allow for individual attention and participation in discussions. The suggested staffing and duties for a Defensive Falls School with approximately ten to twelve participants includes the following:

- Physician–Discuss physiological changes in Parkinson's disease and aging that might increase the risk for falling.
- Psychologist–Discuss cognitive changes that contribute to a risk for falling. Also, discuss physiological changes in Parkinson's disease and aging that might increase the risk for falling if physician is not available. Administer EXIT test.
- Environmental Designer–Discuss built environment and common risks of falling found in most environments.
- Nurses–Discuss transfer techniques, assistive devices. Experienced Parkinson's disease nurses for physical examinations.
- Other assistants–At least three, trained to help administer assessments such as bean counting, upgaze, visual contrast.

Following the initial teaching and discussion session,which lasts approximately one and a half to two hours, individual assessments are done for each participant. The individual assessment portion of the Defensive Falls School is divided into seven assessment areas:

- Fine motor coordination
- Vision
- Balance
- Gait
- Muscle coordination
- Physical examination
- Cognition

Seven "stations" are set up for a falls school, one for each assessment. Staff at each station supervise the assessments and record the results. The assessments listed in Appendix B are used in the NREC Defensive Falls School. Other assessments and scales are also available.

Appendix B

Defensive Falls School Assessments

Fine Motor Coordination Assessment: "Bean Counting"

For this fine motor assessment test, the following supplies are needed:

Two small bowls
Dried beans, approximately one cup
Tablespoon

All of the beans are placed in one bowl. The patient is asked to transfer all of the beans from one bowl to the other bowl using the spoon with the right hand . The participant then transfers the beans back to the original bowl using the spoon with the left hand. A stopwatch is used for timing this task.

The measure of performance is based on the time required to complete the task with each hand. See M. S. Gerrity, S. Gaylord, and M. K. Williams, "Short Versions of the Timed Manual Performance Test," *Medical Care* 31 (1993): 616–28, for more tests of this nature.

VISION: UPGAZE

Measurement of upgaze is simple. The test takes less than a minute and requires a penlight. The person being tested looks straight ahead and then upward as far as he or she can, moving only the eyes, not the head. The light beam, positioned at the same elevation as the pupil, is initially focused on the pupil of the eye. When the eye moves upward, the light beam shines on the eye

(1) in approximately the same spot, or
(2) on the pupil-iris border, midway to the iris, or
(3) on the white part of the eye (sclera).

Movement of only 15° is the greatest risk factor for a fall. See J. T. Hutton, I. Shapiro, and B. Christians, "Functional Significance of Restricted Upgaze," *Archives of Physical Medicine and Rehabilitation* 63 (1982): 617–19.

Measurement of Upgaze

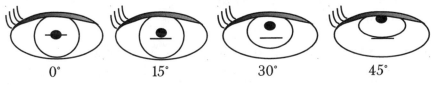

0°   15°   30°   45°

– Indicates light beam

VISION: VISUAL CONTRUCTION TEST

To perform the visual construction test, the participant is asked to copy three simple line drawings using a pencil. The participant is given a sheet of paper divided into six boxes, three above, three below. The line drawings of simple figures appear in the top three boxes. The participant is asked to copy each figure in the box below.

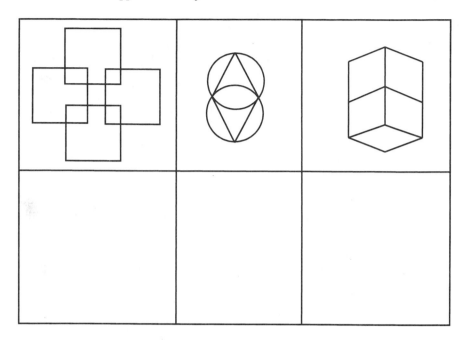

The test is not timed. The accuracy of the copy determines the risk factor. See B. Kolb and I. Wishaw, *Fundamentals of Human Neuropsychology*, 3rd ed. (New York: W. H. Freeman, 1990).

VISION: VISUAL CONTRAST SENSITIVITY

The testing for visual contrast is done using a computerized system that is still considered experimental. However, research in the NREC has shown reduced visual contrast sensitivity with Parkinson's disease that declines with stage of disease.

To perform the test, the participant is seated in a darkened room where he or she can view a television monitor. On half of the monitor are a series of light and dark bars that vary in degree of contrast and in size. On the other half of the screen there is no image. The bars are presented randomly from side to side. The participant is asked to indicate the side of the screen where he or she sees the bars. Contrast sensitivity is evaluated by the computer.

The Neurology Research and Education Center researchers are currently investigating the use of printed wall charts to measure visual contrast sensitivity. See D. Regan, *Regan Low Contrast Letter Acuity Charts Manual* (Sackville, N.S.: Paragon Services, 1994).

BALANCE

The Neurology Research and Education Center uses a computerized dynamic posturography system developed by Nashner and distributed by Neurocom to measure the contribution of sensory organization to balance. By manipulating vision, somatosensory feedback, and vestibular function, the examiner estimates how each of these components contributes to maintaining postural stability.

Balance (postural righting reflex) is usually checked in a clinic setting by a pull test. This method can be used to test balance and righting reflexes in a Defensive Falls School. To perform this test, the patient stands with his or her back to the examiner, making sure the center of balance is established. The examiner tells the patient that he or she will pull backwards on the patient's shoulders on the count of three. The examiner pulls on the shoulders fairly strongly, in an attempt to pull the patient off balance, and observes the patient's ability to regain balance. The examiner is at all times behind the patient and ready to catch the patient in the event that balance cannot be regained. See L. M. Nashner, "Computerized Dynamic Posturography: Clinical Applications," in *Handbook of Balance Function Testing*, ed. G. P. Jacobson, C. W. Newman, and J. M. Kartush (Chicago: Mosby Year Book, 1993).

MUSCLE COORDINATION : PRONATION/SUPINATION

In the NREC Motor Assessment Laboratory, the staff uses a sophisticated computerized system (MOTUS) to accurately measure the degree, speed, and consistency of a ten-second rotation of both wrists. The examiner asks the participant to grip a metal rod that is five inches long and approximately one-quarter inch in diameter. The rod rotates freely in a ball bearing assembly. The participant rotates the rod as rapidly as possible back and forth to the left and right for ten seconds. The test is performed with each hand. The hand and wrist action is similar to that of turning a doorknob back and forth. A small gyroscopic sensor is placed on the back of the hand to measure the activity and translate the results to the computer. The sensor is held in place on the hand with a glove.

If the MOTUS system is not available, the pronation/supination test could be performed as in a regular clinic setting. The examiner asks the patient to rotate both hands back and forth at the wrists, as though turning a doorknob. Slower rotation indicates a lack of flexibility and, for Parkinson's disease patients, indicates that muscles are not working together, but are working in opposition. Fewer rotations and a reduced degree of wrist and arm rotation are predictive of the inability to quickly correct posture on an uneven surface. See J. W. Elias, J. T. Hutton, J. A. Shroyer, et al., "Assessment of Falls Risk in Parkinsonians," presented at International Movement Disorders Congress, Vienna, Austria, 1996.

PHYSICAL EVALUATION

The assessments used for the physical evaluation in the Defensive Falls School are selected specifically for their benefit in evaluating the participant's risk for falling. The assessments for this purpose include a medication history, blood pressure measurement, cognitive function assessment, and the Unified Parkinson's Disease Rating Scale.

Medication History

A complete medication history is obtained for each patient. The examiner asks the patient the following about his or her medicines:

- How long has the patient been treated with levodopa/carbidopa?
- What other antiparkinsonian medications are being taken?
- Are there any other medications being taken for other medical conditions? If so, what medications and for what conditions?

The information obtained from questioning the participant about his or her medications can reveal pharmacological causes for increased risk for falling. Medication side effects and the effects of combinations of certain medications can be pointed out to the patient. If medications are contributing to an increased risk for falls, the patient should discuss the appropriate adjustments of medications with his or her physician. If medication adjustment is not possible, this portion of the evaluation provides the opportunity for teaching the patient about potential side effects associated with the medications. The patient can then be encouraged to take special precautions to avoid additional risks for falls and injury.

Blood Pressure

To assess for postural hypotension, the patient's blood pressure is measured in both the lying (after five minutes) and standing (after one minute) positions. A drop in systolic blood pressure of 20 mm Hg or more is a significant reduction and can produce symptoms such as light headedness or dizziness. Appropriate interventions that the patient can utilize to prevent or decrease a rapid drop in blood pressure are reviewed with each individual who might experience this problem.

Unified Parkinson's Disease Rating Scale

The Unified Parkinson's Disease Rating Scale (UPDRS) is administered by first interviewing the patient to determine how often falls occur, the frequency of freezing, and the frequency of tremor at rest. A healthcare professional trained in performing the motor assessment section of the UPDRS then assesses the following:

Postural stability is a person's response to a sudden posterior displacement produced by pulling or tugging on the shoulders. The individual stands with his or her eyes open and feet slightly apart. The examiner gives the patient instructions to "catch himself or herself" and to avoid falling if possible. Balance is impaired if the patient falls backward or has to be caught by the examiner. Impaired balance is also referred to as poor "postural righting reflex" or "postural instability" and is frequently seen in the advanced stages of Parkinson's disease.

Bradykinesia, or slowness of movement, is assessed by evaluating the degree of slowness, level of hesitancy, and range of motion. Fine motor movements such as turning a doorknob, opening and closing the hands, and finger tapping are tasks the patient is asked to perform to evaluate bradykinesia.

Posture is observed for abnormalities such as stooping, leaning to one side, kyphosis (curvature of the spine so the concavity is backward), and marked flexion (curvature so the concavity is forward). Any one of these characteristics can adversely affect the center of gravity and can result in additional problems with movement and the possibility of impaired balance.

Muscular rigidity is identifiable by the examiner as a sensation of stiffness when moving the patient's major joints with the patient relaxed in the sitting position. Mild rigidity may be activated only if the patient becomes distracted; for example, when answering simple questions or performing a mirrored movement.

Gait is examined for disturbances that may not be evident to the patient. The parkinsonian characteristics of gait are monitored as the patient walks down a hallway. Gait assessment is based upon:

- the degree of slowness of movement
- the presence of small or shuffling steps
- festination (rapid, uncontrolled shuffling)

- difficulty turning around
- decreased arm swing
- the amount of assistance the patient requires while walking

Cognition: Folstein Mini-Mental State Examination (MMSE)

As part of the physical examination portion of the assessment, the Folstein Mini-Mental State Examination (MMSE) is administered. This test measures orientation, registration, attention, calculation, short-term recall, comprehension, reading and writing, and the ability to draw or copy designs. This brief test is given in an interview format and is useful in screening for serious cortical disorders (cognitive problems). See E. P. Feher et al., "Establishing Limits of the Mini-Mental State," *Archives of Neurology* 49 (1992): 87–92.

Cognition: EXIT Test

The EXIT is a fifteen-minute interview that begins by asking the interviewee to continue a pattern of number-and-letter alternation started by the examiner, and concludes by asking the interviewee to describe an object while being distracted. Much of the interview focuses on the ability to stay on task, particularly in the face of a competing behavior or some other form of distraction. Items are scored as follows:

0—the answer is correct
1—the response isn't as clear as it could be
2—the individual misses the item

Scores range between 0 and 50. Executive disability is suspected when scores reach 15 and higher. The higher the score, the greater the disability. Research shows that by stage III Parkinson's disease, about half of those tested have executive function deficits that interfere with daily functioning.

Most individuals with stage IV Parkinson's disease show executive function difficulties. For the examiner to be able to administer and score the test properly requires training; however, professional training in assessment is not required. Any professional healthcare worker could conduct the interview. See D. R. Royall, R. K. Mahurin, and K. Grey, "Bedside Assessment of Executive Cognitive Impairment: The Executive Interview (EXIT)," *Journal of the American Geriatrics Society* 40 (1993): 1221–26; and J. W. Elias, "Normal vs. Pathological Aging: Are We Assessing Adequately for Dementia?" *Experimental Aging Research* 21 (1995): 97–100.

The EXIT and the MMSE are not used as a clinical diagnostic instrument in this context. They are used as a screening instrument to assess one's risk of falling.

CONCLUDING THE DEFENSIVE FALLS SCHOOL

After the assessments of each participant are complete, the Defensive Falls School staff and participants reassemble for evaluation and feedback. At this time, the various assessments are discussed and their purpose explained. The staff members review some of the points discussed throughout the day. The Defensive Falls School participants have the opportunity to ask questions and give input and suggestions of ways to approach the various hazards and falls risks they face daily. Participants are again urged to carefully assess their home environments and make the necessary changes to provide a safe living area.

Appendix C

Parkinson's Disease
Fall Profile©

Name: _____ Date: _____

Stage P.D. _____ Duration of P.D. _____ Years. MMSE Score: _____

EXIT Score: _____

Duration of Treatment with
Levodopa/Carbidopa (Sinemet) _____ Years.

Current P.D. Medications (Check all that apply):

_____ Levodopa/Carbidopa   _____ Anticholinergics (Artane,
    (Sinemet)   Cogentin, Kemadrin, Akineton)
_____ Dopamine Agonist   _____Antihistamines (Benadryl)
    (Parlodel, Permax)   _____Eldepryl
_____ Symmetrel (Amantadine)

Do you take more than four different
prescription meds each day? _____

LIST OTHER MEDICATIONS: _____

_____

Blood Pressure: Lying (after 5 minutes):   _____ / _____ mm Hg
                   Standing (after 1 minute): _____ / _____ mm Hg

Are you dizzy or light-headed upon standing? ____ YES ____NO

Vision: Known eye disease? _____

_____

Visual complaints? _____

_____

Do you have increased difficulty driving at night or dusk?
___YES ___NO

Do you notice that you need brighter light to read or work
with small objects (e.g., handwork, sewing)?
___YES ___NO

Gaze: 0   15   30   45

Acuity _____

Gait: Observe gait on hard surface (tile or wood floor) and on carpeted floor.

UPDRS MODIFIED FOR FALLS RISK ASSESSMENT:

Answer the following items to indicate the patient's status characteristic of the past week:

FALLS:

0 = No falls reported as a result of P.D.
1 = Rare falling, less than one per week.
2 = Occasionally falls, less than once per day.
3 = Falls an average of once daily.
4 = Falls more than once daily.

FREEZING (Sudden immobility of feet) WHEN WALKING:

0 = None or not applicable if unable to ambulate.
1 = Rare freezing, less than once per week; may have start hesitation.
2 = Occasional freezing when walking, less than once per day.
3 = Frequent freezing, more than once per day.
4 = Severe freezing throughout the day.

GAIT/AMBULATION:

0 = Normal.
1 = Mild difficulty. May not swing arms or may tend to drag leg.
2 = Moderate difficulty, exhibiting short steps or difficulty turning, but requires little or no assistance.
3 = Severe disturbance of walking, exhibits festination, propulsion, or freezing necessitating assistance (walker, cane, etc.) at least half of the time.
4 = Cannot walk at all, even with assistance.

POSTURE:

0 = Normal.
1 = Not quite erect, with slight stooping, may be normal for older person.
2 = Moderately stooped, can be slightly leaning to one side.
3 = Severely stooped with kyphosis and/or moderately leaning to one side.
4 = Marked flexion with extreme abnormality of posture.

POSTURAL STABILITY: (Response to sudden posterior displacement produced by pull on shoulders while patient is erect with eyes open and feet slightly apart. Patient is prepared.)

0 = Normal.
1 = Retropulsion, but recovers unaided.
2 = Absence of postural response, would fall if not caught by examiner.
3 = Very unstable, tends to lose balance spontaneously.
4 = Unable to stand without assistance.

BODY BRADYKINESIA & HYPOKINESIA: (Combining slowness, hesitance, decreased armswing, small amplitude, and poverty of movement in general.)

0 = None.
1 = Minimal slowness, giving movement a deliberate character; could be normal for some persons. Possibly reduced amplitude.
2 = Mild degree of slowness and poverty of movement which is definitely abnormal. Alternatively, some reduced amplitude.
3 = Moderate slowness, poverty or small amplitude of movement.
4 = Marked slowness, poverty or small amplitude of movement.

RIGIDITY: (Judged on passive movement of major joints with patient relaxed in sitting position. Cogwheeling to be ignored.)

0 = Absent.
1 = Slight or detectable only when activated by mirror or other movements.
2 = Mild to moderate.
3 = Marked, but full range of motion easily achieved.
4 = Severe, range of motion achieved with difficulty.

TREMOR AT REST:

0 = Absent.

1 = Slight and infrequently present; low amplitude, present less than 25 percent of the day, on average. May not be present every day.

2 = Moderate and bothersome to patient. Present 25–50 percent of the day, on average.

3 = Severe; interferes with many activities. Present 50–75 percent of the day, on average. Patient. must delay some activities due to presence of tremor.

4 = Marked; interferes with most activities. Present most of the day. Patient requires assistance with activities of daily living (eating, dressing, etc.) due to tremor.

MODIFIED HOEHN AND YAHR STAGING:

Stage 0   = No sign of disease.
Stage 1   = Unilateral disease.
Stage 1.5 = Unilateral plus axial involvement.
Stage 2   = Bilateral disease, with recovery on pull test.
Stage 3   = Mild to moderate bilateral disease; some postural insta-bility; physically independent.
Stage 4   = Severe disability; still able to walk or stand unassisted.
Stage 5   = Wheelchair-bound or bedridden unless aided.

Appendix D

Suggested Readings and References

PRACTICAL MANAGEMENT RESOURCES

Atwood, G. W. *Living Well with Parkinson's.* New York: John Wiley and Sons, Inc., 1991.

Carpman, J. R., and M. A. Grant, eds. *Design that Cares: Planning Health Facilities for Patients and Visitors.* Chicago: American Hospital Publishing, Inc., 1993.

Carroll, D. *Living with Parkinson's Disease: A Guide for Patient and Caregiver.* New York: HarperCollins, 1992.

Cohen, A. M., and W. J. Weinter. *The Comprehensive Management of Parkinson's Disease.* New York: Demos Publications, 1996.

Coté, Ron, ed. *Life Safety Code.* Quincy, Mass.: National Fire Protection Association, 1997.

Dauphine, S. *Parkinson's Disease: The Mystery, the Search and the Promise.* Tequesta, Fla.: Pixel Press, 1992.

Duvoisin, R., and J. Sage. *Parkinson's Disease: A Guide for Patient and Family.* 4th ed. Philadelphia: Lippincott-Raven, 1996.

Gordon, S. *Parkinson's: A Personal Story of Acceptance.* Boston: Branden Publishing Company, 1992.

Grist, R., M. J. Hasell, R. Hill, J. L. West, T. R. White, and S. K. Williams. *Accessible Design Review Guide.* New York: McGraw Hill, 1996.

Hutton, J. T., and R. L. Dippel, eds. *Caring for the Parkinson's Patient.* Amherst, N.Y.: Prometheus Books, 1989.

Kataria, M. S., ed. *Fits, Faints, and Falls.* Boston: MTP Press Ltd., 1991.

Lesnoff-Caravaglia, G. *Aging in a Technological Society.* New York: Human Sciences Press,1988.

Lieberman, A., and F. Williams. *Parkinson's Disease: A Complete Guide for Patients and Caregivers.* New York: Simon and Schuster Fireside Books, 1993.

McGoon, D. C. *The Parkinson's Handbook.* New York: W. W. Norton and Company, 1990.

Nissen, L., R. Faulkner, and S. Faulkner. *Inside Today's Home.* 6th ed. Fort Worth: Harcourt Brace College Publishers, 1994.

Pearce, J. M. S. *Parkinson's Disease and Its Management.* London: Oxford Medical Publications, 1992.

Pitzele, S. K. *We Are Not Alone: Learning to Cope with Chronic Illness.* St. Paul, Minn.: Thompson and Company, Inc., 1986.

Shumway-Cook, A., and M. H. Wollacott. *Motor Control: Theory and Practical Applications.* Baltimore: Williams and Wilkins, 1995.

Tideiksaar, R. *Falling in Old Age: Its Prevention and Treatment.* New York: Springer Publishing Company, 1989.

RESEARCH RESOURCES

Bles, W., and T. Brandt, eds. *Disorders of Posture and Gait.* Paris: Elsevier, 1986.

Birren, J. E., and K. W. Schaie, eds. *Handbook of the Psychology of Aging.* 4th ed. San Diego: Academic Press, 1996.

Burleson, L. K. *Parkinson's Disease: Relationship Between Environmental Design and Falls Risk.* Ph.D. diss., Texas Tech University, 1992. Unpublished.

Cummings, S., et al. "Risk Factors for Hip Fracture in White Women." *New England Journal of Medicine* 332 (1995): 767–815.

Elias, J. W. "Normal vs. Pathological Aging: Are We Assessing Adequately for Dementia?" *Experimental Aging Research* 21 (1995): 97–100.

Elias, J. W., J. T. Hutton, J. A. Shroyer, Z. Curry, J. M. Stewart, A. Bednarz, J. M. Schwantz, T. Hutton, J. A. Ribble, and L. Cruz. "Assessment of Falls Risk in Parkinsonians." Presented at International Movement Disorders Congress, Vienna, Austria, 1996.

Elias, J. W., J. E. Treland, J. T. Hutton, P. New, D. Royall, R. K. Mahurin, and J. A. Shroyer. "The Value of Using Brief Assessment Measures for Executive Function As Well As Mini-Mental-State Type Screening Measures." Presented at the Sixth Cognitive Aging Conference, Atlanta, Ga., 1996.

Feher, E. P., R. K. Mahurin, R. S. Doody, N. Cooke, J. Sims, and F. J. Pirozzolo. "Establishing Limits of the Mini-Mental State." *Archives of Neurology* 49 (1992): 87–92.

Gerrity, M. S., S. Gaylord, and M. K. Williams. "Short Versions of the Timed Manual Performance Test." *Medical Care* 31 (1993): 616–28.

Gibson, M. J., R. O. Andres, B. Isaacs, T. Radebaugh, and J. Worm-Petersen. "The Prevention of Falls in Later Life." *Danish Medical Bulletin* 34, supplement 4 (1987): 1–24.

Horak, F. B., J. G. Nutt, and L. M. Nashner. "Postural Inflexibility In Parkinsonian Subjects." *Journal of the Neurological Sciences* 12 (1992): 1–13.

Hughes, P. C., and R. M. Neer. "Lighting for the Elderly." *Human Factors* 23, no. 1 (1981): 65–85.

Hutton, J. T., J. L. Morris, J. W. Elias, R. Varma, and M. A. Poston. "Spatial Contrast Sensitivity Is Reduced in Bilateral Parkinson's Disease." *Neurology* 41 (1991): 1200–1202.

Hutton, J. T., I. Shapiro, and B. Christians. "Functional Significance of Restricted Upgaze." *Archives of Physical Medicine and Rehabilitation* 63 (1982): 617–19.

Jankovich, J., and E. Tolosa, eds. *Parkinson's Disease and Movement Disorders.* 2d ed. Baltimore: Urban and Schwartzenberg, 1988.

Kolb, B., and I. Wishaw. *Fundamentals of Human Neuropsychology.* 3rd ed. New York: W. H. Freeman, 1990.

Nashner, L. M. "Computerized Dynamic Posturography: Clinical Applications." In *Handbook of Balance Function Testing,* edited by G. P. Jacobson, C. W. Newman, and J. M. Kartush. Chicago: Mosby Year Book, 1993.

Pak, H. J. *Perception of Environmental Design Factors Related to Falls Risk Among the Independent Elderly.* Ph.D. diss., Texas Tech University, 1995. Unpublished.

Regan, D. *Regan Low Contrast Letter Acuity Charts Manual.* Sackville, N.S.: Paragon Services, 1994.

Rockstein, M., and M. Sussman. *Biology of Aging.* Belmont, Calif.: Wadsworth Publishing Company, 1979.

Royall, D. R. "Precis of Executive Dyscontrol As a Cause of Problem Behavior in Dementia." *Experimental Aging Research* 20 (1994): 73–94.

Royall, D. R., R. K. Mahurin, and K. Grey. "Bedside Assessment of Executive Cognitive Impairment: The Executive Interview (EXIT)." *Journal of the American Geriatrics Society* 40 (1993): 1221–26.

Tinetti, M. E., and L. Powell. "Fear of Falling and Low Self-Efficacy: A Cause of Dependence in Elderly Persons." *Journals of Gerontology* 48 (1993): 35–38.

Vellas, B., M. Toupet, L. Rubenstein, and L. Christen, eds. *Falls, Balance and Gait Disorders in the Elderly.* Paris: Elsevier, 1992.

Whitney, S. *Patients at Risk for Falls: Quantifying Behaviors and Planning Functional Interventions.* Seminar & Material Sponsored by Northern Speech Services of Gaylord, Michigan, Houston, Tex., 1997.

Wichman, T., and M. R. DeLong. "Pathophysiology of Parkinsonian Motor Abnormalities." In *Advances in Neurology*, vol. 60, edited by H. Narabayashi, T. Nagatsu, N. Yanagisawa, and Y. Mizuno. New York: Raven Press, 1993.

Woollacott, M. H., and A. Shumway-Cook, eds. *Development of Posture and Gait Across the Lifespan.* Columbia: University of South Carolina Press, 1989.

Woollacott, M. H., A. Shumway-Cook, and L. M. Nashner. "Aging and Posture Control: Changes in Sensory Organization and Muscular Coordination." *International Journal of Aging and Human Development* 23 (1986): 97–114.

Youdim, M. B. H., and P. Riederer. "Understanding Parkinson's Disease." *Scientific American* 52 (1997): 52–59.

Appendix E
Contributors

The development and production of the Defensive Falls School, along with the resulting videotape and handbook, was the product of a team of contributors who have worked together to provide a practical and useful guide to prevention of falls. The following people have spent the past three years working on this project.

Angie Bednarz, R.N., B.S.N.
Clinical Research Nurse
Neurology Research and Education Center at St. Mary of the Plains
    Hospital
Lubbock, Texas

Zane Curry, Ph.D. (Editor)
Associate Professor
Department of Merchandising, Environmental Design, and
    Consumer Economics
Texas Tech University
Lubbock, Texas

Jeffrey W. Elias, Ph.D. (Editor)
Associate Director for Research
Sanford Center on Aging
Reno, Nevada

J. Thomas Hutton, M.D., Ph.D. (Editor)
Neurologist
Director, Neurology Research and Education Center at Covenant
    Health System
Medical Director, National Parkinson Foundation Center of
    Excellence
Lubbock, Texas

Trudy Hutton, J.D.
Administrator, Neurology Research and Education Center at
    Covenant Health System
Coordinator, National Parkinson Foundation Center of Excellence
Lubbock, Texas

Judy Ribble
Information Specialist
Neurology Research and Education Center at Covenant Health
    System
National Parkinson Foundation Center of Excellence
Lubbock, Texas

JoAnn Leavey Shroyer, Ph.D. (Editor)
Professor and Chairman
Department of Merchandising, Environmental Design, and
    Consumer Economics,
Texas Tech University
Lubbock, Texas

Janet Schwantz, M.S., CCC/SP
Speech Pathologist
Neurology Research and Education Center at Covenant Health
    System
Lubbock, Texas

Janice Stewart, R.N., B.S.N.
Clinical Nurse Coordinator
Neurology Research and Education Center at Covenant Health
    System
Lubbock, Texas